"*Navigating Trans Voicing* is a stunning book which goes far beyond its remit of enabling speech and language therapists to be gender affirming in their practice. The 50 key points introduce the reader, succinctly and movingly, to the current state of knowledge about sex and gender, as well as to the current state of crisis around transphobic politics and gender-related care. Readers are taken by the hand through reflections on their own genders and voices, and through straightforward, gentle introductions to good practice. The open, vulnerable dialogues between the authors themselves really bring the material to life, and powerfully illustrate the kinds of practices they're suggesting. A wonderful book for speech and language therapists, and for anyone wanting to know more about the current state of gender, how gender relates to voice, and how to work in affirmative ways with trans and non-binary people."
Dr Meg-John Barker, psychotherapist, internationally recognised author of How to Understand Your Gender; Gender: A Graphic Guide; *and* Life Isn't Binary

"Congratulations to Natasha and Matthew on a book that is not only educational but inspiring and thought-provoking. The authors' discussion allows a level of vulnerability for the reader whether they are new to the space or a seasoned professional. With such succinct and vital background to trans health in addition to its core concepts, this is essential reading not only for speech and language therapists but for anyone working with the gender diverse community or even seeking to explore their own authentic expression through voice. Bravo!"
Dr Alison Berner, Speciality Doctor in Adult Gender Identity, President of the British Association of Gender Identity Specialists

"Surviving the storms encountered on your Odyssey across an often hostile socio-political sea and bringing back the Golden Fleece of authentic expression requires a new kind of compass – a paradigm shift. *Navigating Trans Voicing* is such a compass and Lode star for all of us embarking on this voyage."

Annie Morrison, voice therapist and teacher, author of The Moment of Speech

"This is a text which is aimed at student speech and language therapists, those new to the field and those drawn to discovering more about trans affirmative voice work. It is a perfect introduction to the principles and fundamentals of becoming a trans affirmative voice practitioner in the way it breaks down the key issues into 50 easy to digest, bite-sized pieces. Each point is filled with words of wisdom and experience and together they set the scene to give a thorough overview of what it means to be a trans-affirmative speech and language therapist. Thank you, Natasha and Matthew – this book will be of benefit to many as they start their vocal journeying."

Nazlin Kurji-Smith, Clinical Lead in Trans Voice and Communication, Northern Region Gender Dysphoria Service, National Adviser in Trans Voice for the Royal College of Speech and Language Therapy

NAVIGATING TRANS VOICING

This book is a resource for those new to the field of trans voicing. It summarises 50 key points needed to work collaboratively and effectively with trans and non-binary people, covering sections on:

- Trans cultural knowledge, sensitivity and awareness.
- Vocal pedagogy and the therapeutic relationship.
- Fundamental know-how and voice therapy principles and exercises in trans voicing.

Written and developed by both a leading consultant speech and language therapist in trans voicing, and a psychologist and counsellor from the trans community, the book centres a unique collaboration of clinical and lived experience expertise and is deeply trans-affirmative in approach.

Matthew Mills (he, him/they, them) is gay, queer and identifies as cis-liminal. He is Lead Consultant Speech and Language Therapist and Head of the Speech and Language Therapy Service at the largest and oldest gender identity clinic in the UK (Tavistock and Portman Gender Identity Clinic for Adults, London) where he has worked since 2009. He is a National Adviser in Trans Voice for the Royal College of Speech and Language Therapists, and a founder member of the Trans Voice Clinical Excellence Network (CEN).

Natasha Stavropoulos (she, her) is an openly trans female psychologist and therapist. Natasha is a regular educator and trans awareness trainer for speech and language therapists in practice and in training for the Royal College of Speech and Language Therapists Clinical Excellence Network (CEN).

NAVIGATING SPEECH AND LANGUAGE THERAPY

Navigating the field of speech and language therapy can seem overwhelming to students and newly qualified therapists. This series is designed to provide concise, entry-level summaries of key areas in speech and language therapy, providing a basic insight into a specific area of therapy. Comprising practical advice and guidance from an expert in the field, the books cover topics such as assessment, therapy, psychological approaches and onward referral. This is a useful tool for anyone new to speech and language therapy, or building confidence in their field.

Navigating Trans Voicing
50 Key Points to Support Students and Newly Qualified Speech and Language Therapists with Gender-Affirming Voice Therapy
Matthew Mills and Natasha Stavropoulos

Navigating Voice Disorders
Around the Larynx in 50 Tips
Carolyn Andrews

Navigating AAC
50 Essential Strategies and Resources for Using Augmentative and Alternative Communication
Alison Battye

Navigating Telehealth for Speech and Language Therapists
The Remotely Possible in 50 Key Points
Rebekah Davies

Navigating Adult Stammering
100 Points for Speech and Language Therapists
Trudy Stewart

NAVIGATING TRANS VOICING

50 KEY POINTS TO SUPPORT STUDENTS AND NEWLY QUALIFIED SPEECH AND LANGUAGE THERAPISTS WITH GENDER-AFFIRMING VOICE THERAPY

Matthew Mills and Natasha Stavropoulos

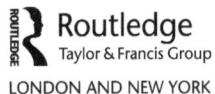

LONDON AND NEW YORK

Cover image: © Getty Images

First published 2025
by Routledge
4 Park Square, Milton Park, Abingdon, Oxon OX14 4RN

and by Routledge
605 Third Avenue, New York, NY 10158

Routledge is an imprint of the Taylor & Francis Group, an informa business

© 2025 Matthew Mills and Natasha Stavropoulos

The right of Matthew Mills and Natasha Stavropoulos to be identified as authors of this work has been asserted in accordance with sections 77 and 78 of the Copyright, Designs and Patents Act 1988.

All rights reserved. No part of this book may be reprinted or reproduced or utilised in any form or by any electronic, mechanical, or other means, now known or hereafter invented, including photocopying and recording, or in any information storage or retrieval system, without permission in writing from the publishers.

Trademark notice: Product or corporate names may be trademarks or registered trademarks, and are used only for identification and explanation without intent to infringe.

British Library Cataloguing-in-Publication Data
A catalogue record for this book is available from the British Library

ISBN: 978-1-032-28923-6 (hbk)
ISBN: 978-1-032-28924-3 (pbk)
ISBN: 978-1-003-29915-8 (ebk)

DOI: 10.4324/9781003299158

Typeset in Aldus
by Deanta Global Publishing Services, Chennai, India

To vocal explorers and gender pioneers building a community of integrity and a world of vocal belonging.

CONTENTS

List of Figures	xii
List of Tables	xiii
Foreword by Barbara Aster	xiv
Foreword by Megan Berrisford-Green	xvi
Acknowledgements	xviii

INTRODUCTION 1

You, the Readers	2
We, the Authors	2
Book Structure and Features	3

Chapter 1
SETTING THE SCENE 5

1	The Non-Binary World of Sex	5
2	The Non-Binary World of Gender	8
3	Starting with *You*	12
4	Terms to Help and Guide	14
5	A Damaging History	21
6	The Harm of Othering	24
7	The Power of Owning	25
8	Author Dialogue 'Under the Microscope'	27

Chapter 2
THE RISK OF VISIBILITY 31

9	Coming Out and Safety	31
10	Transitions and Temporality	33
11	To Name Change or Not to Name Change?	35
12	Author Dialogue 'The Dark Before Dawn'	39

Chapter 3
TRANSPHOBIA AND COMMUNITY RESPONSE 43

13	Widespread Erasure	43
14	Pride and Trans Joy	47
15	Author Dialogue 'The Pearl in the Oyster'	48

Chapter 4
THE ADVOCATE BRIDGE 51

16	Life Commitment	51
17	Why Pronouns?	53
18	Actions Towards Allyship	55
19	Author Dialogue 'Walking with and Taking the Hit'	56

Chapter 5
OVERVIEW OF GENDER-AFFIRMING MEDICAL INTERVENTIONS 58

20	Hormones and Surgeries	58
21	Author Dialogue 'Please Listen to Me'	61

Chapter 6
FUNDAMENTAL PRINCIPLES OF GENDER-AFFIRMING VOICE EXPLORATION 66

22	Vocal Journeying	66
23	Vocal Authenticity	68
24	Vocal Plurality	70
25	Vocal Collaboration	71
26	Vocal Pedagogy	72
27	Therapeutic Affirmations	74
28	Author Dialogue 'Trans Voicing'	74

Chapter 7
THE THERAPEUTIC JOURNEY AND RELATIONSHIP 78

29	Skills and Conditions	78
30	Know the Drama	80
31	Author Dialogue 'In the Boat Together'	83

Chapter 8
ORIENTATION TO GENDER-AFFIRMING
VOICE AND COMMUNICATION THERAPY   85

32	Coaching Ethics	85
33	Your Voice Development in Action	87
34	Your Voice Expansion in Action	89
35	Author Dialogue 'The Sphere and the Cube'	90
36	Motor Learning Principles	93
37	Practical Pedagogy	94
38	How to Coach an Exercise	95
39	Author Dialogue 'Imposter Syndrome to Vocal Belonging'	96
40	The Initial Appointment	98
41	Author Dialogue 'Meeting with the Client'	99
42	High-Bright-Thin Therapy	105
43	Low-Chest-Thick Therapy	110
44	Non-Binary Voicing	112
45	The A + B = C of Practice	113
46	Population Considerations	114
47	Author Dialogue 'Outcomes That Matter'	115

Chapter 9
SUMMARY – THE TRANS-AFFIRMATIVE SLT   119

48	Profession in Crisis?	119
49	Doing the Work: Affirmations and Learning Statements	121
50	Author Dialogue 'Be the Future'	125

Appendix of Resources	129
Bibliography	133
Index	137

FIGURES

1.1	Terms	6
1.2	Charting Privilege and Marginalisation (an Example)	26
6.1	Fundamental Principles Underpinning Trans Voicing Exploration	67
7.1	In Psychological Contact within Voice Therapy	81
8.1	Launch-Express-Land for High-Bright-Thin Voice Work	106
8.2	Low-Chest-Thick (Embodiment) Voice Work	111
9.1	The Trans-Affirmative SLT	122

TABLES

1.1	Potentially Insensitive and Inaccurate Terms	20
5.1	Testosterone HRT	60
5.2	Oestrogen and Testosterone Blockers HRT	60
5.3	Gender-Affirming Surgeries Associated with Medical Transition	61

FOREWORD

Barbara Aster

To begin with, voice is not something everyone thinks of immediately on their journey, in their transition, in their quest – and it is a quest – to become themselves. Maybe the trans person has grown up in or been around the right sympathetic sound environment to pick up and shape a voice they are happy with; most of us have not.

I didn't start to think about my voice until I was being treated in my gender clinic, and then I realised, 'I have to use this voice every day, my voice is one of the main routes people meet me, the way people will know me, even the way people will judge me.' It was a moment! It suddenly dawned on me – I *do* need to work on my voice, to alter it somehow. I don't want that *second look* from someone. Fast forward, and I love my voice. Learning to use it, I have avoided that horrible second look when you get to the supermarket till, or you are ordering a coffee, or you're calling your GP practice.

We are your future clients. We have the tools within us. It is like we are wearing a utility belt with pockets and clips containing our tools and equipment, but we do not know how to use each tool. You, the voice therapist, are there to show us how to use the tools, to help us find what we are comfortable with. You're going to use your voice to help me. You're not going to create a voice for me – you're going motivate me, show and help me unlock the voice that is already here within me, help me *re-find* the colours I haven't used for a long time, the lift, the lightness – whatever that may be for each individual, and if you are working with someone wanting a 'deeper' voice, you're going to help them find strength and solidity in their voice, whether they are taking testosterone or not. And you are going to help people like me build the platform of skill and confidence to use my voice in life situations, in easy, everyday and challenging, dangerous circumstances. Support me, do not be critical of me, do not think I am a figure to be mocked and attacked.

Take a risk with me. Be truthful with me and help me find, practice and enjoy my voice. It's not going to be perfect to the world, but it can be fabulous to me and the people who know and love me, like my beautiful wife, Jen, who supported me and was my rock for 36 years. And while I grieve and miss her desperately – she died during the COVID-19 lockdown – the love, compassion and acceptance she gave me and the vocal play we had together, is in me and I carry that through every day of my life. Jen didn't give up on me. I was seen as me. I was heard as me. I was, and am still loved, as me, for who I am. And I have found the strength to be me, the grit that takes, and it didn't happen overnight and it's something I have to do every day – dig deep, walk proud, be me.

We live in a world where life seems so cheap, a world that needs love. There are as many voices in the world as there are people. Let's create a world where we celebrate each other and speak with whatever voice we have without the judgement, the second look, the violence. You are the voice therapists of a new generation – what you do is so important – study hard, and it will pay huge dividends for your clients and for a world which can speak and sing together.

Barbara Aster (she, her) is a trans woman, and former boxer in early life. She was a care home manager and is now retired. She is a trans awareness trainer for the Metropolitan Police, a regular contributor to LBC Radio, a trainer of speech and language therapists, contributor to a number of clinical books about voice therapy with trans people. She is now a widow; she was married to Jenny for 36 years and their marriage conversion and love story was captured and celebrated in the documentary *The Second Train* by Tellyjuice in 2018.

FOREWORD

Megan Berrisford-Green

The messages in this book brilliantly reflect the years of guidance and training I have benefitted from since realising and deciding, just before qualifying as a Speech and Language Therapist, that I wanted to work in gender-affirming voice. They are lessons I am still learning because cultural humility and vocal discovery are expansive, lifelong processes that cannot be completed as 'tick box' exercises. I encourage anyone drawn to or already working with trans and non-binary people really to take time to read, sense and absorb the wisdom in these pages, knowing that you will be a more skilled and compassionate clinician and human being for doing so.

This book gives you permission to relinquish the role of 'expert' in other people's voices, identities and lives, and invites you to investigate deeply and compassionately your own. It reminds us to open up to our own complexities so we are able to hold and honour the complexities of others. Allow the discussion and practice to shine a light on the myriad of possibilities within your own voice and communication, and to inspire you to uncover things previously unknown to you, for we cannot hope to bring out in others something we have yet to explore and know in ourselves. Above all, I hope this text galvanizes you to stand in solidarity, proudly and visibly, with trans people and make their fight – your fight.

Megan Berrisford-Green (she, her) is a cis Advanced Specialist Speech and Language Therapist at The Tavistock & Portman NHS Foundation Trust Adult Gender Identity Clinic London, and a committee member of the Royal College of Speech & Language Therapists Clinical Excellence Network in Trans Voice. She strives to use her clinical and social privilege to advocate for and collaborate with trans people, and promote equitable access to voice therapy in the health service and through working with trans led community projects.

ACKNOWLEDGEMENTS

We are deeply grateful to the trans and non-binary, gender specialist, voice specialist communities, and their intersections, for their support and feedback during the writing of this text. Particular thanks go to Dr Meg-John Barker (they, them), Jenny-Anne Bishop OBE (she, her), Jane Boston (she, her), Emily Bruni (she, her), Sabah Choudrey (they, them), Sally Collins (she, her), Skye Davies (she, her/they, them), Kaidyn Hinds (he, him), Nazlin Kurji-Smith (she, her), Pam Milman (she, her), Annie Morrison (she, her), Dr Kate Nambiar (she, her), and John Stack (he, him).

Thank you to Sec (he, him) for providing such clean graphics. Thank you to trans and cis colleagues in the European Professional Association of Transgender Health (EPATH), the British Association of Gender Identity Specialists (BAGIS) and the Royal College of Speech and Language Therapists (RCSLT) for their expertise and insight. Thank you to Jane and the team at Routledge for their encouragement and patience.

Above all we acknowledge the lives, stories and legacies of trans, queer and questioning people who have walked before us. We want to express particular gratitude to trans and non-binary people of colour, trans and non-binary elders, and trans and non-binary youth for their courage to dare to be themselves and teach the world that accepting and celebrating each other is the only way to live.

INTRODUCTION

Waiting times for first appointments at gender services for trans and non-binary people are in the region of 23 to 87 months. This is not a misprint. More start-up ('pilot') clinics and smaller gender services are being created to take their place alongside the established and larger gender clinics. The current gender specialist workforce is inadequate in number to support the paradigm shift of colossal referral rates and the scale of unmet client need. The importance of increasing clinical staffing across all multidisciplinary professional groups, including speech and language therapists, cannot be underestimated. There is more interest than ever before from student therapists and newly qualified practitioners to head towards specialising in trans voice. This is indeed welcome, but there are dynamic competencies to grapple with and bed in.

Trans voice is now regarded less as a professional oddity or 'platypus,' the poor cousin to 'proper' medical heavyweight specialisms. There is less of a sense of discounting the field as somehow facile and not serious in relation to core professional training, and a greater recognition and acknowledgment of the nuance it attracts and the skill complexity it requires. The trans voice specialist speech and language therapist must hone dynamic trans cultural sensitivity, engage in personal and deep reflexivity about gender and normativity, have significant skills in voice pedagogy, an experiential felt sense of their own voice through voice training, and robust and responsive therapeutic skills. It is the most politicised area of health care and demands therapists be advocates, and to a certain extent activists, simply by joining the workforce. This book is the beginning of the journey into complexity. Rather than Trans

Voice, we recommend the concept of *Trans Voicing*, because it centres dynamic and ongoing process, plurality and possibility; we mean it as an umbrella term, a queer hug, inclusive of all trans, non-binary and gender questioning people. This book marks an inaugural and unique journey of co-authorship by and intersectional sharing of lived experience and clinical expertise – for the readers' benefit.

YOU, THE READERS

We aim to be useful to you, the student and newly qualified speech and language therapists seeking concise orientation summaries of key issues within this complex field. You may be developing and established specialist therapists and clinicians from other professions reaching for an easy-to-digest introduction and hot topics with experienced guidance.

WE, THE AUTHORS

Matthew Mills (he, him/they, them) is queer, gay and identifies as cis-liminal. He is Lead Consultant Speech and Language Therapist and Head of the SLT Service at The Tavistock and Portman NHS Foundation Trust London Gender Identity Clinic for Adults, where he has worked since 2009. He has over 30 years' experience as a voice practitioner and pedagogue, and originally trained as an actor, singer and pianist at Guildhall School of Music & Drama, and Trinity College London. He is ex officio President of the British Association of Gender Identity Specialists (BAGIS), having served as President 2019–2023. He is a member of NHS England's Gender Dysphoria Clinical Reference Group and a National Adviser for the Royal College of Speech and Language Therapists. He is an HIV survivor of 25 years, a gay rights activist since the 1980s, and advocate and activist for trans rights and social justice.

Natasha Stavropoulos (she, her) is an openly trans female psychologist and therapist, and co-founder of London Gender Support (LGS), a radical gender-centred peer support group in East London. She is a regular trainer for the Royal College of

Speech and Language Therapists Trans Voice Clinical Excellence Network, has contributed to several gender and voice clinical and community texts, presentations at conferences such as the British Association of Gender Identity Specialists, and a documentary on voice by Tellyjuice. She has also given a TEDx talk on personal gender narratives. Originally from Greece, she holds degrees in Computing Science, Digital Design and Animation, Psychology and Counselling, and is currently a counsellor and advocate for clients on a multiplicity of gender journeys and for those living with addictions.

BOOK STRUCTURE AND FEATURES

Fifty Key Points cover a broad range of essential knowledge and skills, and discussion of the contemporary and thorny status quo in the field that a novice, apprentice and journeyperson need in order to expand into a compassionate, effective and trustworthy voice therapist. The text integrates underpinning theory, practical teaching, exercises and questions for mindful reflection, lived experience expertise and guidance, and debate which is not shy of presenting challenge and inviting deep self-interrogation. The book is divided into nine chapters, with varying numbers of Key Points within each:

1. Setting the Scene.
2. The Risk of Visibility.
3. Transphobia and Community Response.
4. The Advocate Bridge.
5. Overview of Gender-Affirming Medical Interventions.
6. Fundamental Principles of Gender-Affirming Voice and Communication Therapy.
7. The Therapeutic Journey and Relationship.
8. Orientation to Gender-Affirming Voice and Communication Therapy.
9. Summary – The Trans-Affirmative SLT.

Some points are pithy and concise, while others are more in-depth, according to their place and import within the discipline.

The text is serious and playful, sober and warm-hearted. It is discursive, unashamedly didactic, sometimes challenging and always supportive. In addition to the co-written text throughout, we include author dialogues at junctures to amplify, clarify and evidence the theory ...

Matthew: As part of the book's features, Natasha, in addition to what we have put forward together in each of the Key Points, we're including dialogues between us. What are we hoping readers draw from these, Natasha?

Natasha: Well, they are further reflections on the themes, the issues, the practice, the politics, the therapy and they are windows into our individual experiences.

Matthew: Yes, in these dialogues the authorial 'we' becomes an 'I' and an 'I' of personal insight.

Natasha: And it is important to say here that while many of the reflections and disclosures are highly personal, we have processed them and they are safe. We are sharing them in a way that is judicious, to facilitate the reader's self-reflection and processing by sharing our own.

Matthew: Thanks for making that clear, Natasha. Yes, these dialogues are not capricious. They are purposeful. We're of course centring the stories and meaning-making from your lived experience and wisdom, Natasha, as someone who is trans; and you also speak from your expertise as a psychologist and therapist, workshop leader and activist; and I offer my insight from my clinical experience as a voice practitioner, teacher and therapist and, where and if pertinent, as a member of the queer community.

Natasha: Our sharing is the tenet of the book. We hope it provides useful and stimulating material to work with and think about. We hope you, the readers, enjoy your learning voyage ...

Chapter 1

SETTING THE SCENE

> **OVERVIEW**
> - This chapter aims to outline the core concepts of sex, gender, cultural humility, positionality, pathologisation, privilege, intersectionality, othering, belonging and owning – see Figure 1.1.
> - It contains Key Points 1–8.

1 THE NON-BINARY WORLD OF SEX

Sex and gender have separate and overlapping meanings and they are far from binary (Barker & Scheele, 2019; Iantaffi & Barker, 2018; Vincent, 2018). We will take these step by step. To begin: sex concerns biology. Sex is all too often assumed to be, and reinforced by the dominant Western cultural discourse as a 'natural' binary of two 'opposites' describing a person as *either* biologically male *or* biologically female. When people talk about sex, they are likely referring to one and/or several components: **chromosomes** (X, Y), **hormone levels** (androgens and estradiol), **genitals** (vagina, labia minora and majora, clitoris, or penis, scrotum, testes), **reproductive organs** (ovaries, Fallopian tubes, cervix, uterus or epididymis, seminal cord, seminal vesicles), and/or **secondary sex characteristics from puberty** (body hair, facial hair, fat-to-muscle ratio and distribution, breast development, height, thyroid prominence, vocal fold length and thickness giving rise to typically perceived voice characteristics).

We tend to take for granted that specific sex attributes coexist and conjoin inextricably with other sex attributes. For

DOI: 10.4324/9781003299158-2

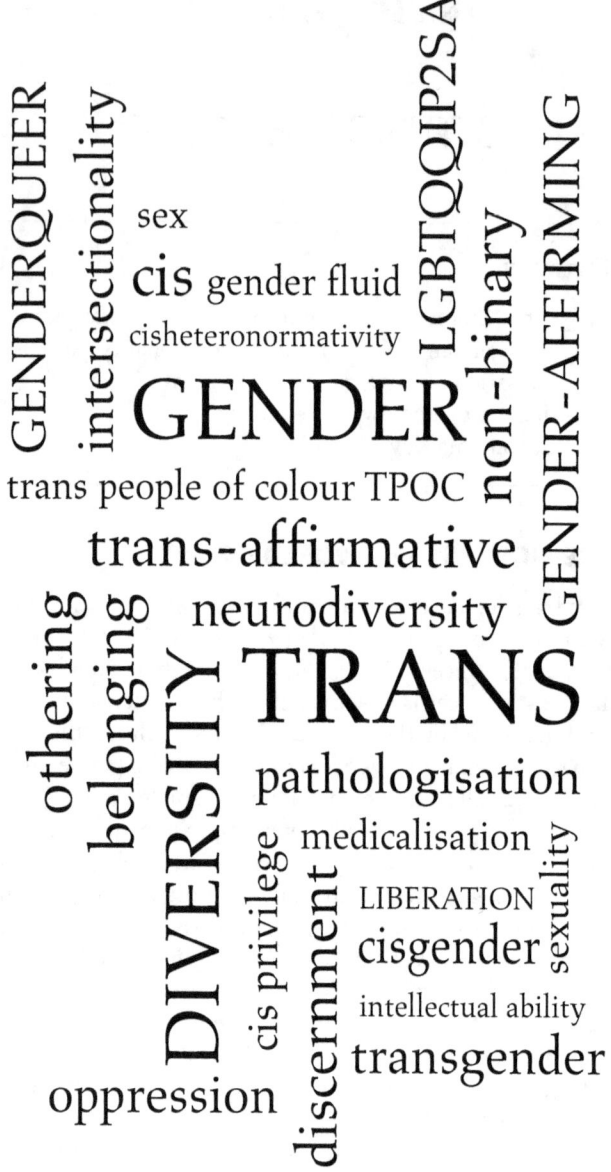

Figure 1.1 Terms

example, females are not females unless they have vaginas, XX chromosomes, wombs, high voices, breast development, smoother bodies, softer skin and are shorter than males who are not males unless they have penises, XY chromosomes, low voices, no breast tissue, hairy bodies, thicker skin and are taller. Sex is also assumed to map onto gender 'automatically'. For example, someone who is sex assigned male at birth due to medically observed and verified genitals of penis and testes is presumed to be a boy, who will become a relatively tall man with a relatively low-pitched voice and a relatively hairy body post puberty in adolescence. In the same way, someone who is sex assigned female at birth due to medically observed and verified genitals of vagina is presumed to be a girl, who will become a woman with breast development, fat distribution around the hips, a relatively smooth body and soft skin post puberty in adolescence.

However – and this is fundamental to your learning – when we interrogate assumption, and examine the degrees of variation that naturally occur, we arrive at the fact that **sex is not binary**. Intersex people, for instance, are people whose anatomy and physiology are not straightforwardly categorised as male or female, observable at birth or emerging during puberty. Intersex people can have chromosomes different from XX or XY, different chromosomes in different parts of the body, and different hormone levels and genital structure from what is expected and regarded as 'usual' or 'normal' by dominant cultures. The 'determinant for sex' has been historically constructed as a medical assessment of genital size deemed performatively adequate for sexual intercourse and procreation in adult life. It is really important to note that the pathologisation and elimination of intersex people through so-called 'corrective' surgeries to make a body conform to standard binary male or female is now illegal in some countries and is a human rights abuse. This kind of genital assessment demonstrates how sex and gender (and indeed sexuality) are bound together by pervasive and unconsciously biased notions of Western sex, gender and sexuality and how a dominant cultural view of binary sex leads to exclusion, harm and trauma for many people (Iantaffi & Barker, 2018).

Not only is sex not binary, there is a vast degree of **sex variation** in human beings such that biological attributes do not map onto others in a rigid or totally predictable occurrence. For example, some people whose bodies are categorised as male without ambiguity are short in height, have little facial hair, significant breast tissue, higher pitched voices and lower levels of testosterone than people whose bodies are categorised as female without ambiguity. Some people whose bodies are categorised as female without ambiguity are tall, have little breast tissue, significantly hairy bodies, lower pitched voices and higher levels of circulating testosterone than people whose bodies are categorised as male without ambiguity. Features we often identify as maleness and femaleness are cultural stereotypes of beauty norms and aspirations reinforced, touted and peddled through advertising, and they are deeply sexist, racist, ageist, ableist, sizeist, etc. (Barker & Scheele, 2019).

2 THE NON-BINARY WORLD OF GENDER

Let us now examine what we understand to be gender. Gender concerns socially constructed categorisations and the multiple meanings and manifestations that flow from them. Notions, judgments and value systems about gender visibly and invisibly shape our sense of who we are consciously and unconsciously, and become deeply ingrained in our psychosocial experiences from the moment we are born. As sex is assumed to refer to a binary of whether someone is biologically male or female, gender is assumed (unless you have welcomed gender diversity in yourself or someone else) to be a binary of whether someone is socially a man and behaves/presents in masculine ways **or** whether someone is socially a woman and behaves/presents in feminine ways. Because of dominant cultural narratives and constructions, we often think of gender as something fixed and predictable and that there are 'normal' and 'natural' ways to identify. But inherited assumption has a snowball effect, and the 'weight of history' sits behind and steamrolls acceptable notions of gender into the present, reinforcing evaluative judgement of how we can experience and express ourselves 'legitimately'. However – and you are engaging in this re-examination of assumption – when we begin to question and know ourselves as unique and utterly individual, the porousness of social construction is realised, and the diverse possibility models of human experience of gender are gloriously revealed.

When people talk about gender, they are likely referring to one or several components. **Gender identity** is a person's entirely unique, personally verifiable sense of themselves (as a boy, girl, man, woman, non-binary person and so on). **Gender expression** refers to the consciously or unconsciously performed behaviours in a social context which form a collection of gender cues from voice, non-verbal communication, choice of attire, pronouns, self-chosen descriptors. **Gender experience** is a person's lived experience of themselves and how they relate intimately to their gender and how they navigate the perception of other people. It especially describes the degrees to which people feel congruent, dysphoric and euphoric with their gender, whether their gender feels stable, changeable, multiple, absent and/or fluid through their life. Gender also includes wider aspects such as **gender roles** (culturally specific domestic, parental, familial, professional roles), and **gender social norms** which are the expectations and stereotypes of the dominant culture about how men and women *should* be, *ought* to feel and are *expected* to behave (for example – degrees of rationality, emotional empathy and expression and so on).

You realised it! As with sex, **gender is not binary**. Barker and Iantaffi (2019) and Barker and Scheele (2019) guide us to understand gender as a myriad of experiences. There are people who experience aspects of their gender which align with social norms, traditional expectations and stereotypes and are comfortable being perceived as 'typically' masculine or feminine. There are people who experience themselves as binary but are androgynous and express themselves in non-traditional ways, rejecting stereotypical gender roles and norms associated with their gender identity. There are people who experience themselves as non-binary and have a gender identity which is between, betwixt and beyond a masculine-feminine dichotomy. 'Non-binary' may refer to an identity in and of itself, in addition to being an umbrella term of gender identities outside a typically described and majority experienced binary system of gender. Certainly, non-binary genders are not a phenomenon of the twenty-first century. Many cultures contain a rich history of gender systems of more than two categories. There are the Hijra or Kinnar of South Asian countries including Pakistan, Bangladesh and India. The Hijra were considered sacred until British colonisation deeply stigmatised them as a 'criminal tribe' in 1871 and, despite legal recognition by the Supreme Court of India in 2014, they continue to be the subject of widespread discrimination and violence. There are the 'Two Spirit' traditions of indigenous people of North America – many tribes have more than two genders, each with specific names and roles which cannot be conflated into one homogenous 'third gender' categorisation. Also, there are the rich traditions of the Mahu in Hawaii, the Fa'afafine in Samoa and the Machi of indigenous peoples in Argentina and Chile, to name a few. Many non-binary identities of these cultures have spiritual, ceremonial and shamanic roles and statuses, and combine and/or move between and/or beyond cultural notions of femininity and masculinity. Many cultural traditions experience gender trauma and have been distorted and ferociously erased from history and common knowledge by the violence of cultural dominance and colonisation because these diverse identities challenge and trouble cisheteronormative views of hegemony (Iantaffi, 2020; Marshall, 2020). Davies urges us to interrogate harmful misconceptions about non-binary people as not experiencing gender dysphoria/euphoria, being 'less certain' than binary trans people, expressing only neutrality/androgyny, and identifying as non-binary because it is 'fashionable' or a 'stepping stone' towards binary identity (in Scarrone Bonhomme et al., 2023, pp. 68–69).

Many trans people are conscious of their gender identity early in life and how it does not align with their sex assigned at birth. Many cis people also question and grapple with traditional meanings of gender and their gender identity, and some experience gender liminality (Mills & Pert, 2024). Furthermore, gender is not separate from but intersects with our many overlapping identities and degrees of social privilege and oppression including race, sexuality, class, nationality, disability, faith and geography. This is *intersectionality*, the work of civil rights advocate Kimberle Crenshaw (1989). Effectively, our identity is always about having *more than one* identity at a time, and our particular identities must be interrogated in relation to patriarchy, white supremacy, colonialism and capitalism as the forces which define, include and exclude identities and bodies as superior or inferior and less valuable and deserving of social rights, resources and privileges (hooks, 2000). It is important to remember that multiple experiences of inequality compound disadvantage and create complex obstacles which can go unnoticed, unacknowledged and not understood by those with relative social privilege. The experiences of a white trans woman will be very different from a trans woman of colour, for example, and we need to be alive to how we may unwittingly erase someone's experience by the assumptions we make. It may be obvious to say this, but we all have to work at how we practically break down the barriers in ourselves and in our environment which exclude people because they have marginalised identities (Faye, 2021; Miles, 2020).

We have aimed to present the cornerstones and complexities of sex and gender and how they are deeply interrelated. In fact, it can be helpful to think not of 'sex and gender' but 'sex/gender' (Fausto-Sterling, 2012). This means we best understand ourselves and each other within a *biopsychosocial* framework of influence, cause and effect. It is not possible to separate our brain and body from our experience of gender, and the gender messaging that bombards us throughout life. Our body and brain development are both influenced by and influence our psychological experience of gender and our relation to social norms and expectations, and degrees of comfort therewith.

We want to touch in to how our sexuality also deeply intertwines with our sex/gender. There is much to explore here, the granular detail of which, with apologies, we do not cover in this text. Go further into this and consult Barker and Scheele (2023) and Iantaffi et al. (2018). Start with yourself – who you are, how you identify, and how you are in your body, and then sense and add in your sexuality. Sexuality, like gender, is a matter of your own personal experience and identification – there is no test for being a man or being gay, for example, no assessment to figure out if you are gay enough to be *gay*, or man enough to be a *man*. So, begin with your sense of your sex/gender and then tune into sexuality, remembering that your sex/gender is who you go to bed *as*, and your sexuality is who you go to bed *with*, as it were.

At the heart of these first two topics is the imperative that neither sex nor gender are binary, that gender is not ever 'just' a matter of biology, and perspectives which define gender only in relation to biology are fearful and reactive constructs of a dominant culture which deny and erase the fact of human diversity in general and gender diverse people's experiences in particular. Once you embrace, straightforwardly, that your genitals do not define your gender, you are well on your way to being a trans-affirmative clinician and a mindful, compassionate human being.

3 STARTING WITH *YOU*

It is largely expected that clinically focussed textbooks begin with discussion of categorisation, then set out assessment criteria for diagnostics proceeding to diagnosis and treatment. This is hypothesis testing in the medical model and fits pathology-based healthcare very well. When working with a population (remembering that no one is ever homogeneous), we need to transform cultural competence into cultural humility which emphasises learning about *ourselves* in relation to population-specific cultural identities and practices. Practically, this means we do not stop at interrogating the concepts of sex and gender, but we examine our own identity and relationship to our sex and gender.

When working with Deaf people, and we identify as a hearing person, we learn sign language taught to us by people who are Deaf. When working with people who stammer, and we identify as someone who is speech-fluent, we need to own our fluency, and learn about what is important to a person who stammers, and centre difference not defect (Campbell et al., 2019). When we offer voice therapy and work with trans and non-binary people, we examine our motivations and do not assume a cisgender vocal superiority. Trans voicing is not about rescuing trans people to become cis acceptable. Some trans people may seek to blend socially such that they are not misgendered on account of their voice; 'passing' may be a desire expressed by some clients, but should never be a term initiated on the lips of a cisgender speech and language therapist due to the social privilege and power weighted towards cisheteronormativity intrinsic to the cis-therapist position (see Key Point 4 below). Therefore, we must drill down into the assumptions that arise from our own identities, our sense of gender, our sense of what gendered voice means to us and to general perception, and how we perform our gender and vocal gender in the contexts of our lives. What is invisible to us remains assumption that leaks out and potentially causes harm to and deletion of the client's personhood, experience and expertise. What is not admitted to or made explicit by we who have clinical privilege cannot easily be challenged or pushed back against by our clients (Mills & Pert, 2024; Mills & Stoneham, 2021).

Below are reflexive questions which require time and space to think about, absorb and respond to. Be mindful and gentle with yourselves. Notice the impulse to skip through or pass by. We invite you to be with the questions; a desire to avoid may mean you do not yet understand the power you hold in clinical and social contexts, and how hurry-up narratives are so much part of capitalist life pressures which tend to discount personal rhythm and investment in self-reflection. Self-understanding provides the experiential raw material to develop your cultural humility, and that is something special and exciting.

- What deeply motivates you to working with trans and non-binary people?

- How do you know yourself to be who you are?
- How do you know yourself to be the gender you are?
- What words do you use to describe yourself?
- What words do other people use to describe you?
- How much does your gender and sexuality need to be explained to people?
- Have you felt diminished or excluded by others on the basis of your gender or sexuality?
- Do you feel very different in your sense of self now compared to five years ago? Imagine yourself in 20 years' time – will you be the same person then?
- Do you seek to 'fit in' or are you your own person, a rule bender and/or rule breaker?
- Can you tell by appearance who is cis and who is trans? Should it matter?
- How do you value yourself?
- How can you value people with different lived experiences to your own?
- How has it been to reflect on these questions?
- What will you do differently in your clinical and social life as a result of reflecting on these questions?
- What title would you give to the story of your development in this field so far?

For further work, look at Bornstein (2013) and Owl and Fox Fisher (2021).

4 TERMS TO HELP AND GUIDE

During training courses we have facilitated, we often notice worry or overwhelm on the part of participants in meeting and using an array of new terms. It is absolutely OK to be unsure and consciously aware of what you do not know at the beginning of your journey towards cultural humility – a dynamic process of ongoing learning. Noticing our anxiety about getting things wrong or offending people are signs that we *do* care and what we say *matters*. So, acknowledge your intention to make a helping relationship. Language is not preserved in aspic but is constantly and mercurially changing. Uniquely discovered, freshly minted, intimately personal, language tells the stories of our lives – the words that sing, the talk that hopes, the fabric of endurance, the celebration of relationship (Denborough, 2014). There are many ways people describe themselves, differences in and between groups. Owl and Fox Fisher remind us that 'some people grew up in a different time and find solace in words we might deem outdated nowadays' (Fisher O & F, 2021, no pagination). Our clients will use language which fits them and it is not our place to 'correct' people with lived experience, but join them in mutual understanding.

Therefore, terms are not 'out there', but, rather 'in here' – in us and with us. We offer brief definitions and discussions of pertinent terms below, as well as suggestions of ones to avoid. Behind every phoneme, every morpheme, every term, live individual people with unique tales of intersectional resilience and emergence, whom we witness and honour with our engagement right here and now.

Assigned at birth – indicating how someone's sex/gender was assigned and presumed by medical observation of the genitals at birth and registered on the birth certificate – e.g. 'assigned male at birth' (AMAB), 'assigned female at birth' (AFAB).

Affirmative – having an affirmative stance means that we celebrate the whole person. No intervention or surgery can avow or affirm something that is intrinsic and personally verifiable by the individual alone. When we speak of gender-affirming surgery or gender-affirming care, we mean care that enables the person to experience a reduction in their gender dysphoria and a greater sense of gender euphoria and well-being – i.e. it is not the gender that is being affirmed, it is the whole person who is being witnessed and supported. We tend to speak of **gender-affirming** in relation to care, interventions, therapies and surgeries, and

trans-affirmative in relation to the attitudes, behaviours and practices of individuals, clinicians and organisations. A 'trans-affirmative speech and language therapist' is someone who is informed about and sensitive to trans culture, and who actively engages in ongoing self-enquiry about their own cultural position related to cisheteronormativity in their development as an effective clinician, advocate and ally.

Cis (short for **cisgender**) – someone whose gender is congruent and fits the sex they were assigned at birth ('cis' in Latin means 'on the same side' – i.e. the gender aligns with the sex assignment at birth).

Cis-liminal – some cis people experience their gender occupying a space between being cis and trans.

Deadname – many (but not all) trans people change their name related to aspects of their social transition. The deadname refers to the name given at birth or in infancy. It is a big no-no and antithetical to being trans-affirmative for clinicians and administrative staff to use a client's deadname. Doing so will trigger someone's gender dysphoria. Proceed in a way that is trauma-informed (Scarrone Bonhomme et al., 2023). Practically, when writing to the client, in the absence of an official name change by deed poll, we use the client's official name at the top of the letter ('RE:... '), and add the client's name in use in parenthesis. We use the client's name in use throughout the body of the letter or correspondence. Note that a person's name they have in current use is not 'preferred,' it *is*. When we meet someone for the first time, we simply ask 'what would you like me to call you?' or equivalent. There may be many reasons why people are taking time to make an official name change – it is a very personal process.

Gender dysphoria/euphoria – dysphoria is a medical term (not a formal diagnosis) referring to the anxiety and distress experienced by many (though not all) trans people due to the incongruence between their gender and the sex they were assigned at birth. People have very individual experiences of the intensity of physical dysphoria, vocal dysphoria, social dysphoria. Gender euphoria refers to people who have a sense of joy and well-being related to their gender.

Gender Incongruence – 'a marked and persistent incongruence between the gender felt or experienced and the gender assigned to birth' – is the current diagnosis name (*HA60*) in the *International Classification of Diseases,* 11th edition (ICD-11) and has moved from the 'mental and behavioural disorders' chapter into a new 'conditions related to sexual health' chapter. Crucially, trans and gender diverse identities are not mental health conditions and are no longer categorised as pathology. Inclusion of Gender Incongruence as a diagnosis in the ICD-11 enables trans people to access gender-affirming healthcare and health insurance.

Man – trans or cis – a trans man is a man with a trans history (assigned female at birth); a cis man is a man with a cis history (assigned male at birth). Both trans and cis men are straightforwardly *men.*

Misgendering – an act which mistakes someone's gender or assumes their gender incorrectly based on aspects of someone presentation, by naming them wrongly, using incorrect pronouns and descriptors, categories and adjectives. Misgendering can be non-deliberate and a genuine slip-up; more seriously it is a micro- or macro-aggression intending to reduce, shame, dehumanise, invalidate and, more and more in current times, annihilate a trans person and their experience. Any act of discrimination related to someone's trans identity is transphobia, and it is illegal in the UK under the Equality Act.

Non-binary (sometimes written as *'NB',* or *'enby'* and is synonymous with **genderqueer**) – refers to a gender in and of itself as well as being an umbrella term for people whose gender is beyond, betwixt, between and outside the simplistic man-woman/masculine-feminine dichotomy – e.g. **gender-neutral** and **agender** people have no gender; **androgynous** people are somewhere between masculinity and femininity; **bi-gender** and **genderfluid** people may move between genders during their life-time; **pangender** people have plural gender experiences; **third-gender** people experience themselves as having a further gender; **genderfuck** people challenge and trouble the socio-political dominant culture narrative of binary systems including gender.

Passing – means that a trans person (particularly a binary trans person) is perceived socially as the gender with which they identify. It is **never** a term that should be used by a cis person. Indeed, it is deeply unethical and cis-centric to occupy a position of unacknowledged cis privilege in relation to the trans person where, consciously or subconsciously, a cis-assessment of how 'cis enough' a trans person is thought to be is set up by an individual cis person or a group of cis people. Many trans people have goals to 'pass' or 'blend' – and the trans-affirmative clinician will help the client reduce gender dysphoria in contexts and code-switches. Even when your client uses the term 'passing', it is vital that the person's identity is valued in and of itself as authentic. There is no othering, no failing. If you are cis, it is important to be upfront and explicit with your trans client: 'as a cis person, I don't and can't use the word "pass", but I understand when you say that, you mean you want to live and enjoy your life fully as yourself' or equivalent.

Queer – originally a slur, this is a term reclaimed and used not only by many trans and non-binary people, but many LGBTQQIP2SA (Lesbian, Gay, Bisexual, Transgender, Queer, Questioning, Intersex, Pansexual, Two-Spirited and Asexual) people. Its meaning evokes identities and practices which oppose normative structures and categories. 'It is a wormhole through the structure and temporality of cisheteronormativity, creating and expressing its own framework, qualitatively independent of normative system and categorization. It rejects, is vocal and visible, and stands politically proud. It gives *the finger*' (Mills & Stoneham, 2021, p. 36). Like all identifying names and labels used by marginalised people, minority groups and sub-cultures, describing oneself as 'queer' can only be done by the person, not by others. Naming by others is a presumption: it robs people of their personal experiences and potentially weaponises them.

Trans (short for **transgender**) – someone whose gender is not congruent and does not fit with the sex they were assigned at birth ('trans' in Latin means 'across' – i.e. the gender does not align and is across from the sex assignment at birth).

'Trans' or 'Trans and Non-binary'? – many non-binary people describe themselves as trans, and some do not. We refer to people as **trans and non-binary people** to mean that everyone is trans, but acknowledge that some non-binary people experience themselves within the trans umbrella term and some do not. Our reason for explicitly referring to 'and non-binary people' comes from discussions with many non-binary people who argue for greater non-binary visibility in social, political and linguistic terms.

Transfeminine – someone who is assigned male at birth and identifies more with femininity than masculinity, and may include binary trans women as well as non-binary people.

Transmasculine – someone who is assigned female at birth and identifies more with masculinity than femininity, and may include binary trans men as well as non-binary people.

Woman – trans or cis – a trans woman is a *woman* with a trans history (assigned male at birth); a cis woman is a *woman* with a cis history (assigned female at birth). Both trans and cis women are straightforwardly *women*.

Table 1.1 outlines terms we suggest are best steered away from because they are mostly considered inaccurate, outmoded, salacious or judgmental.

Ultimately, we celebrate our clients with the language they use because they are experts in their lives, and there is absolutely nothing to rectify.

Table 1.1 Potentially Insensitive and Inaccurate Terms

Steer away from	Because	Use instead
sex change	centres sex over gender assumes a trans person was not their gender all along is headline grabbing	gender dysphoria
tranny	is a slur fuels sexual violence	trans man trans woman trans person
transsexual	is outdated centres medical diagnosis and pathology	trans man trans woman trans person
transman/ transwoman/ transpeople	'trans,' like 'cis,' is a separate word and adjectival (only use 'trans' when it is absolutely relevant and the person has given consent)	(trans/cis) man (trans/cis) woman (trans/cis) people non-binary person
Male-to-Female (MtF)/ Female-to-Male (FtM)	assumes a history of identification emphasises transition history over current identity	trans woman trans man non-binary person
natal/born male/female	ignores the crucial process of assignation at birth centres sex over gendered body	assigned male at birth assigned female at birth
real/normal/ natural	is transphobic to imply a trans people are not real invalidates non-binary people	men women non-binary people
transgenders	is inaccurate: 'trans' is an adjective not a noun it erases other identity aspects and is othering	trans people (most people say 'trans' rather than the more formal 'transgender' but 'transgender' is OK)
biologically male/female	centres genitalia at birth implies biology governs gender invalidates gender experience as an individual process	[trans/cis] man [trans/cis] woman [trans/cis] people non-binary person

We leave you with Juno Roche who writes in *Trans Power*:

> Using the word 'trans' alone ... stands up proud, it's radical and bold in the face of attack and in the face of gender demands. It provides a comfortable space for others to grow up in without needing any words – perhaps future lives without labels. 'Trans' alone is a finger up to gender expectations and limitations. The word 'trans', as a destination, has the capacity to truly shake the patriarchal structures to the ground ... Trans as a destination is aspirational ... Transness really is a new space ... a spacious truth.
> *(Roche, 2020a, p. 255)*

5 A DAMAGING HISTORY

This is a charged section, so we give a trigger alert here. Breathe out and take time to absorb what follows and let it settle within you gently.

Embarking on your journey to meet and work *with* trans and non-binary people means you need to know and constantly hold in your mind the significant history of medicalising and pathologising trans people which casts long shadows of trauma into the present. Trans people have been viewed through a cis-centric lens in healthcare for more than a century. Not very long ago, trans people were viewed as **sexual deviants** and people with **identity disorders**. Diagnoses applied to trans people from the World Health Organisation's *International Statistical Classification of Diseases and Related Health Problems* (ICD) have been 'Transvestitism' in category 'Sexual Deviations' (ICD-8); 'Transsexualism' in category 'Sexual Deviations' (ICD-9), 'Transsexualism' in category 'Gender Identity Disorders' (ICD-10). The American Psychiatric Association's *Diagnostic and Statistical Manual of Mental Disorders* (DSM) retains 'Gender Dysphoria' in the DSM-5 (2013) but is categorised as a mental disorder. The ICD is used in the UK. Importantly, in 2018, the ICD-11 redefined gender-identity health with 'Gender Incongruence of Adolescents and Adult' and 'Gender Incongruence of Childhood' which have been moved out of category 'Mental and Behavioural Disorders' into a new chapter dedicated to 'Conditions related to Sexual Health.' This shift represents 'current knowledge that trans-related and gender diverse identities are not conditions of mental ill-health, and that classifying them as such can cause enormous stigma' (www.who.int/standards/classifications/frequently-asked-questions/gender-incongruence-and-transgender-health-in-the-icd).

Despite no longer being categorised as having a mental disorder, trans people are still often required to jump through invasive assessment hoops steeped in cisgender bias to 'prove' how trans they are, and ready for treatment. Non-binary people often report feeling straight-jacketed to present a more 'acceptable' binary history. It is important to know that there still exists a fear of gate-keeping approaches where clinicians take overall responsibility for deciding who gains access to which treatment. Moreover, clinical assessments related to commencing hormones or referring for surgeries have historically been carried out with very little cultural sensitivity or respect for lived expertise. Gladly, the architecture of assessment has substantially changed and is now more collaborative and responsive to the client, but clinicians need nonetheless to own the power they wield in the clinical space, and build bridges of trust and respect with the trans community (Lorimer & Vincent, 2022). Necessarily, assessment and diagnosis lead to access to care. For a useful discussion of the arguments for and against assessment see Richards and Barrett (2021). Most especially, there is a rich tapestry of lived experience accounts – we recommend deep diving into Sabah Choudrey (2022), Travis Alabanza (2022), CN Lester (2017), Christine Burns (2019), Chelsea Manning (2022), Juno Roche (2020b), Finn Gratton (2019) and Janet Mock (2017).

When we add in the NHS crisis of wait times, especially in gender services which at the time of publication averages a 5-year wait for a first appointment at a gender clinic and 13 months between subsequent follow-ups (for hormone and surgical referrals), the trans client experience is dismaying. In addition (see also Chapter 3), there currently exists a political and social climate characterised by widespread dehumanisation and denial of trans rights, and culture wars which perpetuate narratives that gender is a matter of biology, that being trans is a pathology, that trans ideology removes rights from women, that trans people require conversion 'therapy', and young people who are gender-questioning and seeking to explore or make steps to socially transition, trigger a safeguarding referral. Cultural opposition to all things trans is now affirmed and applauded in political life at the highest level, despite the fact that politicians are neither experts nor clinicians in the field, and there is semantic drift which describes approaches to trans care now as 'exploratory' rather than 'affirmative', which is in fact not-so-thinly veiled transphobia. The gender critical movement has capitalised on biased and inaccurate, often sensational, press coverage of young and adolescent trans people's services, where language of 'experimentation' and 'children' have been crystallised in the minds of some of the worried general public, such that people little noticed when the Court of Appeal *overturned* the High Court judgment that trans adolescents did not have competence to give consent for puberty blockers.

There are some positive steps, in that new gender clinics and services are emerging within the NHS, created with more collaboration with the trans community and third sector organisations (charities, voluntary groups and social enterprises) supporting trans people. This is welcome, *but* we need to build a new generation of sensitive and effective clinicians at ease with gender diversity, committed to self-reflection, and in solidarity with the trans, non-binary and queer community. We end this point on a sober note. There is deep concern among gender specialist clinicians that the NHS's 'early adopter' services (primarily involving Alder Hey Children's NHS Foundation Trust in Liverpool and Great Ormond Street Hospital in London) to replace the Gender Identity Development Service for young people and adolescents are woefully ill-equipped to meet current and projected demands. Problems with recruitment of adequately specialist clinicians, with staff training programmes, and deep divisons in treatment approach have created significant delays to opening these new clinics. All the while, young people and their families have been largely ignored throughout this crisis. There is a high prediction of failure regarding these new services, which will inevitably increase the plight and despair of those most vulnerable seeking compassionate care at the centre of this debarcle.

6 THE HARM OF OTHERING

We cannot un-know Key Point 5; therefore, we proceed by scrutinising two powerful human processes – the defence of *othering* and the emotional intelligence of *owning*. We issue another trigger warning further to what follows. Read, pause, focus on your breathing, let it be soft, and continue. We start with permission to think the unthinkable and listen to those thoughts unheard and denied in the margins of ourselves; we modify cognitive distortions and harsh reactive judgements through conscious relationship.

In states of high arousal and hypervigilance, under physical or socio-emotional duress, we default to the reptilian brain reactions of fight, flight, freeze and faint – strategies to move us out of imminent danger and preserve life. We are hard-wired to spot difference – that which stands out from the accepted and expected, that which might be predatory. What we perceive as unfamiliar is often characterised as 'out there', 'not part of me', 'not part of our group', and we erect an 'us and them' dynamic which literally makes people *strange, alien* and *other*. When we feel robbed, attacked and terrorised, we close ranks, ossify membership, generalise and exclude on the basis of identity characteristics – *those trans people, the gays, the migrants in boats*. In counter-defence and assertion to be seen, we also tend to split category membership into such tiny pieces that would, in logical conclusion, render us all othered and annihilated. Moreover, the creep of invalidating people judged unacceptable by the dominant group is ramped up by the current existential crisis of climate change, threatened resources, harrowing war and conflict, unprocessed grief for the enormous losses of place, people and species, information addiction and overwhelm, the march of potentially dehumanising technology, and our increasing inability to think critically and discern with compassion. When we deny our common humanity, we create a culture of uncare – this is the process of ***othering***.

The antidote is to develop radical trust and embrace our fear of the unknown. Seeing and being seen, hearing and being heard make us feel that we are valued and that we belong – sharing with each other the individual stories of our lives of hope, struggle and emergence. When we foster self-interrogation over complacency, response over reaction, connection over isolation, and solidarity over guilt and conflict, we create belonging communities founded on the premise that the circle of existential concern includes all humanity and all life, where behaviours which denounce, devalue and dehumanise are given no oxygen.

7 THE POWER OF OWNING

Think of how a camera lens is able to widen the field of view and hone into a single sharp focal point. This is analogous to the mechanisms of sight and hearing and how we process information. The psychological process of **owning** is similar and centres self-efficacy: focusing inward, investing in ourselves and our knowledge base, and focusing outward, being accountable and taking responsibility for what we know, do, believe and understand.

Working out what we believe in and stand for – separating out what we can claim as truly our own and what has been internalised from family, teachers, religious leaders, politicians and authority figures – is the process of developing an informed position. It is a muscle we learn to flex through training, supervision, meditation, psychotherapy. Being a therapist necessitates that we make conscious our identities and the power we have in a clinical (and social) space. Being mindful of implicit biases, social programming and assumption, is taking ownership and developing our *positionality*.

Privilege manifests as a system of bestowed rights, benefits and advantages automatically accessible to a dominant group alone. We do nothing to deserve or seek these special treatments and statuses – they come with particular aspects of our identities due to how social hierarchy is and has been constructed. Privilege is mostly not consciously experienced: its power and jurisdiction become visible and felt only when curtailed, endangered or removed. Privilege without insight gives us the option to *decide not to see* a disadvantaged person or group.

Figure 1.2 is a schematic *example* of how social privilege and marginalisation manifest across a number of identity categories. There are many further identities (for example, handedness, body size, neurodiversity, language, accent, parental status, intellectual ability, etc.) not included here, but you can use the basis of this example and add in more categories important to you. Use the diagram to review how privilege and

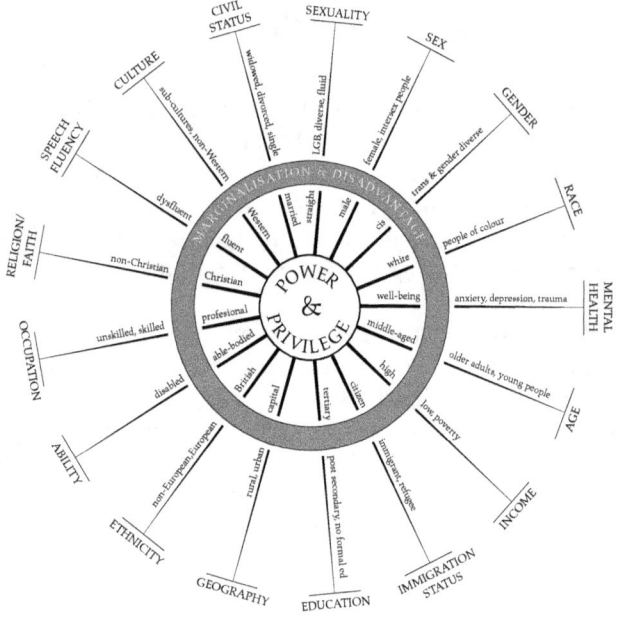

Figure 1.2 Charting Privilege and Marginalisation (an Example)

oppression presents in your life. Consider situations where you have progressed with ease – without question or barrier. Reflect on scenarios where you have felt judged, ridiculed, shamed and been denied access. If you travel through the world as cisgender and heterosexual, these being perceived as fitting more 'standard' social expectations and attracting greater privilege, the full force and influence of cisheteronormativity is likely to be invisible to you. This is cisgender privilege. It is essential that we know how we relate to cisheteronormativity so that we do not reduce gender diverse people into that construct. It can feel uncomfortable, even painful or shameful, squaring up to our privilege. We may feel guilt conceding that features of our identity have given us, whether we like it or not, power over other people. Acknowledging our position means we have a standpoint and we make space for people, we listen to their struggles, we speak out about social inequities and advocate for social change and the dismantling of oppressive systems.

8 AUTHOR DIALOGUE 'UNDER THE MICROSCOPE'

Matthew: We have introduced some big themes in this first section, Natasha.

Natasha: We have – setting the scene, preparing the ground, a lot to look at under the microscope.

Matthew: Yes, understanding that sex and gender are not binary. Examining new terminology. Such helpful steering from you, thank you.

Natasha: The most important starting point to inform your developing practice is knowing that trans people, LGBTQ people widely, have historically been pathologised – by professionals who intended to be harsh and by those who intended to help but have operated within models of pathology. Trans people don't require pity about this; we want clinicians to affirm us. That means you straightforwardly listen and believe what we say about ourselves. Yes, trans healthcare is better today but there are still practices which persist in denying our validity and legitimacy, and in categorising us as deviant and mentally ill.

Matthew: Yes, it's not a facile start. Knowing how trans healthcare has developed and what state it is in now is fundamental to being a therapist who can give the best service to trans people today.

Natasha: We are all in progress. We all need to do *the work* of gaining knowledge and understanding, challenging our assumptions. The theme of self-examination of our position and status as people and clinicians runs through every part of this book.

Matthew: Thanks, Natasha, for centring this for us.

Natasha: It is so important right now when we see such extreme right wing political and societal views that call for the annihilation of trans ideology and the violent rejection of trans people. Every day, trans and non-binary people are written and spoken about as people who are deluded, confused, fraudulent; we're trouble-makers, objects only of sexual fetishism, imposters, perpetrators of sexual violence and people whose existence takes away the rights of others. This is a very challenging time to be trans. And being trans is not a choice.

Matthew: It's deeply worrying. We're going to talk more about transphobia and hate crime in Chapter 3.

Natasha: Yes, certainly. What is happening in the current political climate is all the more reason that we reach out to the reader as experts from lived experience and clinical experience and say – use your intelligence, use your compassion. These discussions come from people who know first-hand. Please do not be seduced by implicit biases that damage all of us. Making people bad and conceptualising people who are different as freaks and unwanted is really damaging to all of us, to our common humanity. Thank you for not othering people. Let people be themselves. It takes nothing from anyone else.

Matthew: We are working to know the filters that colour our perception, because as professionals we have power weighted towards us.

Natasha: Matthew, yes. We are asking the reader – please don't make your professional status and ambition trump your ethics and de-value trans people. Don't proclaim your expertise about us and about our voices when you might only have a perfunctory relationship with us, or worse, when there is no trans person consulted with in your claims. We hope you, the reader, take seriously our request to think about your gender – it's all part of the work required.

Matthew: This is a huge subject and deeply personal, but I wonder whether you might say something about your own gender journey, Natasha?

Natasha: Yes, of course. Well, I guess I consider myself to have been born into a body which expressed male biological features, which I then transitioned into a female body. My gender identity transcended that body, it transcended that maleness, since my gender was always female/woman as I understand it now, retrospectively looking back. I couldn't express this when I was very young, but now I realise that I was always female/woman in my gender and psychologically, and that transcended my male body as it was assigned at birth.

Matthew: And how do you respond to references in the press about 'realness' related to men and women? What might you say about this?

Natasha: It's not helpful. It's reductive and actually transphobic. Gender identity transgresses the limitations of the body. It's beyond physicality. It's a totally false binary to think of gender as 'real/not real.' Gender is. Cis or trans, your gender is as you experience it. The biopsychosocial aspects of gender and identity are unique and complex for everyone. The personal, psychological aspect must be respected – I mean that gender is personal and self-verifiable, how I feel, how I see myself, how I define myself even if externally I present differently or atypically to expectation. Also, gender can be fluid and not fixed for many people. We can grow into and mould ourselves into presenting in ways that we are happy with. And that can change from day to night and from here to there. So, gender is, in my experience not static, but rather dynamic in essence. And you, Matthew, describe yourself as cis-liminal – can you say something about this?

Matthew: Thank you for these deep insights, Natasha. Yes, for me, cis-liminality is about occupying a space between being cis and being trans. I have not transitioned, but in the course of my life I experience myself as increasingly liminal and fluid, and I use pronouns which are mostly he, him, and sometimes they, them.

Natasha: It is important for everyone to realise that we are all human, and that at some level we might all think of ourselves as trans in that we all have the potential to experience change in our gender identity.

Matthew: Thank you for sharing parts of your journey, Natasha. These are not matters to invite voyeuristic curiosity.

Natasha: No, we have chosen to speak about personal aspects in a processed way as a way to encourage the reader to look through the lens of their microscope into their relationship with gender and normative programming.

Matthew: Thanks, Natasha.

Natasha: By being transparent we hope to motivate the reader to make their implicit biases conscious, to develop a compassionate and thought-out position. Then voice work can happen without fear of judgment.

Chapter 2

THE RISK OF VISIBILITY

> **OVERVIEW**
> - This chapter aims to outline the core concepts of coming out, stealth, transition, trans-temporality, transphobia, transmisogyny, transmisogynoir, cis-sexism, name change, Gender Recognition Act, Equality Act.
> - It contains Key Points 9–12.

9 COMING OUT AND SAFETY

Coming out is a metaphor describing a person's decision and *action* to self-disclose about their gender identity, sexual or romantic orientation, or physical or mental health status which will bring a sense of joy, euphoria, but also feelings of shame to be released. Coming out may be *implicit* by giving names or pronouns, or *explicit* where a story is revealed and shared. It can refer to a single event, but is invariably a multifaceted and multiplot process over the course of someone's life. Coming out can feel like a psychosocial 'death' and 're-birth' with all the significance these words invoke. The first, inaugural, coming out is usually the most potent in risk, and the person claiming the marginalised, stigmatised identity – trans, gay, HIV positive, for example – is at the point of desperation, expecting total rejection and social annihilation. Think about what struggle for the most basic survival must be present in the face of expecting utterly to lose loved ones, friends, family, partnership, marriage, children, companionship, community, intimacy, social welcome, job, professional standing, career, housing, finances, care, love, belonging. It is a fight for life, that if not done, despite the enormity of anticipated and actual loss, would lead to self-harm, self-decline and suicide. There are millions of lived accounts from people who have indeed experienced loss at this scale many times over.

However, what is *gained* is life, resilience and self-reliance to rebound and reshape in the face of adversity. Think of a time when you have had to make sacrifices or compromises in favour of pursuing a life path of greater personal authenticity. When we align with our deepest values, we set off on a voyage into the unknown, and decide what to take with us, and what to leave behind that we can or may no longer carry. These may be provisions, resources, qualities, identities, relationships or attitudes. These journeys and thresholds are archetypal rites of passage to be celebrated, not diminished or weaponised, as we listen and witness them. Again, self-examination means we respect stories without influencing people who are deciding how they wish to be for themselves. People decide to come out in specific contexts relative to degrees of safety and the need to disclose and self-protect.

Trans people experience discrimination, simply by virtue of existing, and physical and emotional violence from societal objection to diverse identities (Alabanza, 2022). Trans women and transfeminine people are subject to misogyny, known as *transmisogyny*, sexism known as *cissexism*, and transphobia. Trans women of colour are subject to intersectional oppression of transphobia, misogyny and anti-blackness – known as *transmisogynoir*. Ashlee Marie Preston is a trans woman of colour and has written powerfully on 'The Anatomy of Transmisogynoir' (see www.harpersbazaar.com/culture/features/a33614214/ashlee-marie-preston-transmisogynoir-essay/). Non-binary and transmasculine people also experience erasure, and some or all of those prejudices and pressures arise from a toxic masculine 'legitimacy'. Living as an 'out' gender diverse person is challenging, and their intersectional identities of race, class, ability and so on, deepen the complexities and hurdles of day-to-day existence.

Some trans people live 'stealth' or 'in stealth' which means they choose to disclose their gender history to no one, or to very few trusted people within their social milieu. This selective non-disclosure of someone's trans status can literally mean the difference between staying alive or not, as there are many situations in which being visibly trans attracts discrimination, abuse, violence and murder. From a safety perspective, if a trans person, in their terms, is able to 'pass' socially with their gender expression, living in stealth protects against unwanted sexual attention and potential fetishisation, and indeed may open up social and professional opportunities often not available to an openly trans person. However, living in stealth is psychologically harmful as it reinforces social and personal invalidity – not feeling or being seen and heard as someone's true self. However, more and more, living in stealth and not coming out is the safer option for a trans and non-binary person attempting to exist in an increasingly intolerant and transphobic world.

10 TRANSITIONS AND TEMPORALITY

Gender transition is defined as the time point, or, dynamically, several time points, when a trans person makes deliberate changes to their gender expression in order to fit with their gender identity in a way which potentially expands life possibilities and allows them to live fully and comfortably as themselves. Crucially, transition is not about becoming a man, woman or non-binary person, but rather 'about becoming oneself and making one's peace with that decision' (Richards & Barker, 2013, p. 41). Aspects of transition may or may not be dependent upon another, and can be undertaken in holistic, discrete and/or separate stages. Gender journeys and transitions are dynamic processes: people morph, change, adapt and align multiple facets of self-hood in growth and evolution. As we discussed in Chapter 1, gender can be experienced as fluid and emergent by both trans and also cis people. A gender timeline may or may not be linear according to typically observable stages of development. Social 'arrival' checkpoints and rites of passage may well occur at a different physical age for some trans and non-binary people compared with their cis contemporaries. For example, a young trans person may experience the onset of unwanted puberty in typical early teenage adolescence but be unable to celebrate an adolescence which fits their identity both psychologically and physiologically until they have embarked on hormone replacement therapy (HRT) in, perhaps, their late teens, early- or mid-twenties. Similarly, a middle-aged trans person may enjoy a late experience of youth in their social and intimate life related to psychological readiness and, largely, better access to health care currently, compared to lower levels of personal resilience and health care provision when younger. This phenomenon is known as **transtemporality** (Pearce, 2018). Further, some binary trans people may shape-shift into more non-binary identities and expressions at different stages of life, and vice versa. What is important to understand is that we must guard against bringing an expectation that transition temporality will always occur in parallel with a typical cis trajectory of stages of psychosocial development and emergence. This is highly relevant in the context of exploring voice and code-switching. No assumptions can be made about how and when people become themselves: it is an ongoing process and every day is a new day as ourselves, just as every day is a new 'beginning' with our voice. We are in a constant and evolutionary state of *becoming*. Transition timelines, and the nuance of how people identify and express across time and space, are diverse and need to be supported and celebrated in their own right (Faye, 2021).

There are different kinds of transition. **Social transition** (sometimes called social role transition) involves taking steps to living authentically in a person's affirmed gender. This may include any one (but not necessarily all) of the following – self-disclosing a trans identity to family members, friends, partners, colleagues at work, school mates, teachers, fellow students at college or similar; making changes in appearance and behaviour (clothes, personal grooming/style, voice); using a name, a set of pronouns and styles of address which are congruent; making legal changes to name and registrations. Social transition can subdivide into *occupational* (specific employment and HR processes related to transition in the work place); *educational* (transitioning at school, college or university); *vocal* (stepping into using a voice, voices, or codes which fit with social and intimate contexts); *spiritual/faith* (being open about transition related to someone's spirituality to leaders/co-members of a religious or spiritual/faith community). For young people, social transition means the child is able to participate in family, school and other activities in accordance with their gender identity, including being introduced to peers and adults using the name and pronouns that affirm the child's stated gender. Likewise, social transition for trans and non-binary adolescents needs to centre the young person's expertise in their life, and we must listen to their needs.

Social transition can be just one part, or even the whole of a trans or non-binary person's transition journey. It can precede or follow a **medical transition**, which involves taking hormones and undergoing life-affirming surgeries. Essentially, it is harmful and reductive to think of transition as simply meaning 'swapping' one role or category to another in a binary way. A non-binary transition and a binary trans transition proceed in a way particular to the individual's needs and readiness, supported by clinical services which work to international clinical standards and guidance (World Professional Association of Transgender Health's Standards of Care 8, 2020) and national service specifications (NHS). There is no right or wrong way to be trans or non-binary, and there is no right or wrong way to transition.

11 TO NAME CHANGE OR NOT TO NAME CHANGE?

An important part of social transition, yet not one that every trans and non-binary person will opt for, is a legal name change. 'In the United Kingdom, a change of name is easily done and carries enormous legal, symbolic, and emotional significance' (Richards & Barrett, 2021, p. 93). Name change can be **straightforward for some and complex for the others** who may need wider support from the gender clinical team through counselling psychology to help them through this. It is vital to note, as we emphasise in Chapter 1, that trans and non-binary people do not *ever* require mandatory psychotherapy for being trans and non-binary, and *trans-ness* is not a mental condition. However, gender services provide counselling if the client chooses and needs more time to reflect on aspects and directions of transition. Gender services are still grappling with what 'non-binary social transitions' look like, and there is a great deal of work that gender clinicians have to do to acknowledge cis binary unconscious and conscious biases around binary gender categories of name and name change. Au fond, the client needs to understand the challenges and ramifications of pursuing name change or not.

Below we set out some of the details regarding name change, offered not to encourage voyeurism but in the spirit of strengthening the multidisciplinary approach to clinical work. A change of name deed or Deed Poll (downloaded free of charge with no requirement to instruct a solicitor) enables a legal name and is witnessed by two adult British citizens who are non-family members. A statutory declaration is essentially the same except that it has to be witnessed by a solicitor or notary public and there is a fee for this service. Once the Deed Poll is completed, the new name can be registered with a new sex marker in institutions and associations such as health care providers, dentists, banks, utility providers, loan companies, employers, universities and colleges, the electoral registry, HMRC, the council, health clubs, societies and more. The Deed Poll will facilitate removal of reference to the deadname on commercial databases (telecoms companies, gym memberships and so on). These change processes can be long and tiresome, and usually do not happen overnight but can take up to a year or more to complete.

- **Name** – changing name is a deeply personal statement of identity and one which will transmit some information to other people, but we must be careful not to make judgements around the name choices people make, however quirky or non-contemporaneous they may seem within a normative bias.

- **Styles of address** or British social titles (Ms, Mr, Miss, Mx, Mrs) – should not be confused with *titles* (Dr, Professor, Lord, Dame, etc.), also referred to as nobility, academic or religious titles, which denote rank, training and social privilege. Social titles carry no rank and can be used without a deed poll change. Many non-binary people and some binary folk use 'Mx' as a neutral style of address.
- **Registrations** – changing name and sex markers on NHS records is possible with the Deed Poll. Once a new NHS number is issued, all medical information should be transferred to the new record and there is no link to the old record within the new one. Qualification documents and certificates can be changed to the new name via the examination board or registration body.
- **Driving licence and passport** – the DVLA and Passport Agency will change name but will only change sex marker with an accompanying letter of confirmation by a medical practitioner or psychologist that the person is living in their affirmed gender and that the change is likely to be permanent.
- **Gender Recognition Certificate (GRC)** – the Gender Recognition Act (GRA) (HMSO, 2004) provides that a UK GRC changes legal sex status to one other than that was assigned at birth. It is 'awarded' by a Gender Recognition Panel within the Appeals Directorate of the Judiciary. A person needs to have lived in their affirmed gender for two years, often dated from the Deed Poll, and provide a report from a gender dysphoria specialist as part of this administrative process. There is no requirement for a medical transition to have been undertaken.
- **Birth certificates** – someone can change their gender marker ('M' and 'F') on their birth certificate with a GRC.
- **Non-binary legal gender status** – none exists at present. This is deeply regrettable. In the 2018 consultation to review the GRA, 58% of respondents called for non-binary gender legal status; in 2021, the British government

rejected a further petition for non-binary gender legal recognition, reporting no plans to extend or review the GRA.
- **Marriage** – The Married (Same Sex Couples) Act 2013 makes no requirement for trans people to require a GRC to get married but the ceremony wording would treat the couple as if they are same sex, even if they are not. Holding a GRC means the person can opt for marriage or civil partnership.

The Gender Recognition Act (HMSO, 2004) is important in that it confers legal status for the binary trans person. It is, however, viewed as problematic as it is effectively an administrative body seeming to rubber-stamp someone's gender, which by definition, is personally verifiable only. There are calls for a legal system to be adopted based on self-identification with necessary checks and balances. The Gender Recognition Act Reform 2022 was voted in by the Scottish Parliament lowering the minimum age for applicants to 16 years, moving away from psychiatric diagnosis and medical evidence to statutory declaration, and reducing two years lived in role to three months, in line with international best practice. At the time of writing, however, the British government has lodged a Section 35 which blocks the bill from gaining royal assent.

The Equality Act (HMSO, 2010) lists gender reassignment as a protected characteristic, making it illegal to discriminate on the basis of someone's trans status. The GRA (HMSO, 2004) and the Gender Recognition Order (HMSO, 2005) render it an **absolute illegal offence** to disclose that a person is trans if this information has been gathered or transmitted in your professional role *without* the trans person's **consent to disclosure**. This means whichever health service you work in, you must ask and record the trans person's consent to disclosure to other health care professionals (and you need to be specific which ones and what the purpose is). We return to the essential theme that 'trans' is an *adjective* to be used only when pertinent, relevant and consented to. It is a criminal act to 'out' or disclose a person's trans status without their expressed permission when the trans person holds a Gender Recognition Certificate (Richards & Barrett, 2021; Vincent, 2018).

12 AUTHOR DIALOGUE 'THE DARK BEFORE DAWN'

Natasha: Obviously, the risk of being authentic and being yourself, when that is variant in some way relating to gender – well, the risk is *transphobia*. The problem is transphobia. It's the programming in society that tells people that it's ok to be horrible to trans people in the way people behave towards us, the way people react to us, the way people deny us love.

Matthew: Yes.

Natasha: That is the risk of being visible. And for some trans people, especially trans women of colour in certain parts of the world, this risk means the risk of being physically attacked, of losing one's life, of being murdered. The greatest risk to oneself. And for those of us who can weigh up that risk, and feel able to be seen – and yes, heard too – the benefit to being visible – and audible – is that we create a *precedent*.

Matthew: I think that is such an important word and concept – precedence, creating a precedent. It's a kind of a paradigm shift, in a way.

Natasha: Yes, absolutely. We create a 'possibilities model' as Laverne Cox describes it. We create a possibilities model of how to exist in a way that feels authentic and is variant in some form or other, and for that to be OK, to feel ok, to be myself, my own glorious variation. There are as many possibilities as there are people, and I can express myself in the way I want to. I don't want to hide my *Transness*, and personally I locate myself in quite a binary trans way, but I don't want to lie to anyone about me being trans. So, I am openly trans, like many of us who risk being open, and this creates a very real precedence.

Matthew: Walking together in risk and being seen.

Natasha: Yes. It was something that 20 years ago and further back, people in my position didn't have as an opportunity, most people lived in stealth, because the world – hard to believe it – was even more transphobic than it is currently, despite the daily threats of violence and erasure that trans people meet today. The world then was even less accepting of gender variance, so you had to hide, we had to hide. It is still not accepting now and hate is rife – we are going to discuss this in the next section.

Matthew: So, there is greater visibility of and for trans and non-binary people now, but it seems very heavy and deeply worrying that we live in times which are so oppressive to trans and queer people, and many marginalised groups, with a relentless pursuit and barrage of opposition expressed as fear narratives from a challenged patriarchy.

Natasha: Absolutely it is. It is relentless. From the top echelons of society downwards.

Matthew: I was really moved at the recent 8th BAGIS symposium in Cardiff, two eloquent, brave young transmasculine people aged 17 and 18, stood before an audience of nearly 200 delegates, and spoke from the heart and told of their strength and unshaking clarity about knowing themselves, being openly trans and adolescent, and how painful it is for them, at their young age, to read every day the stories of hate and destruction towards trans people – as one said – 'that's me you're writing about and I am 17 and I have my whole life in front of me, and I am not confused about who I am and I am not going away.' They received a standing ovation. Incredible young people. But what challenge and struggle at the beginning of their lives.

Natasha: Yes, amazing resilience. There's that expression, that saying – *the darkest part of the night is just before the break of dawn*. It gets darker before it gets brighter again. I think I agree with that, and hold on to hope with that. Because of social media, because people feel able to share strong opinions, many even feeling it's ok to incite violence, things that people are now being open about, venting about, commenting on – these things can be harsh, ignorant and hateful.

Matthew: Yes, bad behaviour and bad mouthing takes place and is acted out in plain sight now – in the media, in politics, leaders who lie in plain sight, we know who they are, and it's accepted as OK. The world has skewed and fragmented into a sense that 1 + 1 rarely equals 2 now, but 1 + 1 now equals 2.4 or 1.7, as it were, in terms of people being unable to think critically and question the denial, the bluff, the deceit and acts of aggression that are expounded, heard, witnessed, entered into and accepted as how things are and the status quo of the now-normal. An outpouring of the shadow of humanity.

Natasha: Yes, an outpouring of the shadow, that's a great way to put it, and so right, because we are ultimately talking about states of consciousness of human beings and our evolution towards becoming more compassionate, more accepting of the diverse ways to be human, letting go of the need to other, to oppress, to control and destroy those who don't conform to a majority standard, and are perceived as threats to territory and resources that belong only to the dominant group. And yes, everyone feels braver in front of a keypad or keyboard and feels empowered and enabled to express strong opinions which affect other people directly even if those views are overtly transphobic or racist or prejudiced in some form. We've lost accountability, and people feel even less accountable online, and, as you say, also now in plain public view.

Matthew: And not just *hiding* in plain sight, as yesterday's strategy of those in power abusing power for personal gain, but now one step further – being openly prejudiced, supported and 'celebrated' for being so in plain sight. But despite all this, you believe, Natasha, that there is benefit in being visible, being gender warriors and brave explorers as Juno Roche says, and setting precedence.

Natasha: I do, and of course it is a mix of very personal factors that have allowed me the *privilege* of being visible – the loving support from my family, for example, which unfortunately is still a relatively rare or ambivalent occurrence for many. Trans people often have to find new families, queer families, where queer bond is definitely greater than blood tie, because it has solidarity and love and acceptance. But my blood family support, and my queer family support and that from my friends, as well as the unconditional positive regard and affirmative stance of my gender specialist clinicians, my therapists, my voice therapists – all these have enabled me to accept myself at a core level *enough* to want to be visible, to not hide my *Transness*.

Chapter 3

TRANSPHOBIA AND COMMUNITY RESPONSE

> **OVERVIEW**
> - This chapter aims to outline the core concepts of minority stress, macro- and micro-aggressions, hate crime, moral panic, culture wars, conversion practices, Trans Joy, Trans Day of Remembrance, Trans Day of Visibility, Pride.
> - It contains Key Points 13–15.

13 WIDESPREAD ERASURE

We begin this chapter with a trigger warning. It is sobering. We have given quite an amount of space here to emphasise the extent and intensity of the problem. You would have needed to have been sequestered on a desert island not to be aware of the current culture war about trans identity. Trans identities are discounted as not real and there is an insistence based on public ignorance and unconscious bias that gender (as well as sex) is a matter of biology alone. In attempts to pursue their own agendas and careers, politicians, including the most senior in the UK, have indulged in openly transphobic comment with no clinical expertise or nuanced understanding of the field. Not all, but most of the press coverage about the Gender Identity Development Service was sensationalised and inaccurate, and stirred up moral panic around trans adolescents characterised as inferior to cis adolescents in Gillick competence and understanding of themselves. Gladly, this High Court judgment was overturned by the Court of Appeal, though press reporting of the latter was given considerably less national profile than the former. Further to the oppositions to trans identities, there has been no ban of conversion practices aimed at gay and trans people, despite government rhetoric for five years. Cat Dixon, Chair of Stonewall, issued a statement:

> We are deeply disappointed to see that legislation to ban conversion practices has been dropped from the King's Speech. This was the final opportunity for this UK Government to protect LGBTQ+ people from the abuse and torture that has afflicted generations of LGBTQ+ people in the UK and which continues to this day.
> *www.stonewall.org.uk/about-us/news/ stonewall-statement-uk-governments- failure-ban-conversion-therapy*

At the 8th Scientific Symposium of the British Association of Gender Identity Specialists (BAGIS), the council and membership agreed to publish the following statement in response to the Conservative government's call to disallow trans women into female wards in hospitals. The statement was read out in front of 200 delegates and gained a standing ovation in solidarity with the trans community:

> BAGIS statement on equal access to healthcare. *6th October 2023.*
> The British Association of Gender Identity Specialists (BAGIS) asserts the rights of all people who are eligible to receive healthcare in Britain, to do so without fear of discrimination and hatred. Recent attempts in British society to remove the access of gender diverse people to their equal right to healthcare appear to be solely in the pursuit of political gain. The BAGIS condemns the use of gender diverse people to further political careers and agendas.

We call on healthcare workers to continue to provide high quality care as is their duty and, almost without exception, also their desire. We offer our allegiance to our gender diverse service users, colleagues and friends in healthcare and our assurance that we see the harm that the recent political statements have caused. We call on politicians of all parties to seek to protect the human rights of gender diverse people and speak out against those who seek to spread transphobic bigotry and hate within our healthcare system.

https://bagis.co.uk/bagis-statement-on-equal-access-to-healthcare/

The relentless transphobia experienced by trans people in the UK and world-wide is of deep concern. Moreover, there are individuals who call for the annihilation of trans people and those who treat trans people. Meyer's *Minority Stress Model* (1995) explains the chronic stress, anxiety and depression people with marginalised identities experience as a result of the stigmatisation they are subjected to on a daily basis. Trans people are predicted to have significantly poorer physical and mental health, and significantly greater suicidality than cis people related to their internalised transphobia, sense of shame, and social and structural exclusion (Bockting et al., 2020). Dealing with the impact of minority stress can lead trans people into drug addiction and substance misuse, depression, anxiety and a range of other mental health challenges. We need to work in a trauma-informed way and create supportive policies and programs that address the needs of trans individuals, and work to reduce factors that perpetuate shame and stigma.

Misgendering, harassment and violence against trans and non-binary people take many forms. They can be visible or invisible, and perpetuated consciously and subconsciously. Transphobia – from Greek *phobos* – means fear of trans people, the expression of which can be casual, insidious and layered. It is always damaging. Discrimination often occurs in work, health care and housing settings. Micro-aggressions can occur as accidental misgendering, questioning someone's identity or gender expression, making assumptions about someone's gender, silences on the phone, an eye roll, a double-take and being specifically or generally disbelieved. Macro-aggressions are altogether more serious and involve the intention to cause harm to a trans individual, by inciting physical and/or mental violence through intentional misgendering, and by enacting verbal and physical abuse, and assault. These types of aggressions essentially characterise trans people, especially trans women as imposters and perpetrators of sexual violence. Macro-aggressions aim to exclude trans people from taking an equal, active part in society, and lead people to feel totally rejected, fearful and unsafe. Trans hate crime is the most serious form of discrimination and occurs as transphobia combined with racism, sexism and misogyny. For the avoidance of doubt, there has never been a case where a trans woman has entered a women's toilet in order to abuse or rape cis women. Read *The Gender Wars and Difficult Conversations about Trans* (Barker & Ryan-Flood, 2023). In forensic settings, there have been men convicted of rape who subsequently attempt to claim a trans identity by way of manipulating their forensic environment and sentencing; such individuals are not trans.

According to Stop Hate UK the trans community is the most targeted group in the LGBT+ community:

> In 2020/2021, 2,630 Hate Crimes against transgender people were recorded by the Police, an increase of 16% from the previous year (Home Office, 2021). This number is still severely underreported because out of 108,100 responses to the National LGBT Survey, 88% of transgender people did not report the most serious type of incident. 48% of transgender people were not satisfied with the Police response after reporting the most serious types of incidents.
>
> *www.stophateuk.org/about-hate-crime/sexual-orientation-and-transgender-identity/*

According to the 2021 *Trans Lives Survey* conducted by TransActual UK:

- 40% of respondents reported having experienced transphobia when seeking housing.
- 63% of respondents reported experiencing transphobia while seeking employment, rising to 73% of respondents who were Black people and people of colour (BPOC).
- 85% of trans women reported being subjected to transphobic street harassment from strangers, with 71% of trans men and 73% of non-binary people saying the same.
- 69% of BPOC respondents reported experiencing transphobia from their line manager at work, and reported consistently higher rates of experiencing transphobia from colleagues (88% compared to 73% of non-BPOC).
- 80% of non-binary people reported having experienced transphobia from colleagues compared to 73% of trans men and 73% of trans women saying the same.
- 99% of trans people surveyed have experienced transphobia on social media.
- 93% of participants reported that media transphobia had impacted their experiences of transphobia from strangers on the street.

transactual.org.uk

14 PRIDE AND TRANS JOY

The trans community, despite many odds stacked against it, is robust, resourceful and exemplary in creating supportive, inclusive and queer spaces in which to meet and find **Trans Joy**. Cis clinicians can also celebrate and centre Trans Joy through our work, which means not only enabling clients to experience an alleviation of gender dysphoria, but also to touch and enjoy tangible periods of euphoria in being trans. We who are cis can celebrate Trans Joy as part of being human in a world that ceases to other and diminish people.

There are a number of important cultural landmarks which are deeply important to the trans community. The Trans Day of Remembrance (**TDoR**) is commemorated on 20th November each year. It is a memorial and candlelit vigil for all those trans people, particularly trans people of colour, who have lost their lives related to transphobia, violence and murder each year. It is shocking and moving in equal measure. We recommend you attend a specific community ceremony. The International Trans Day of Visibility (**TDoV**) is celebrated on 31st March each year, though some members of the trans community feel less comfortable with trans visibility being celebrated as a single-day event, rather than an overall societal acceptance all year. Also, *Trans Pride* marches and gatherings are full of celebration and solidarity. There are a number of cities now hosting a Trans Pride event – London, Brighton, Bristol, Nottingham, Manchester, to name a few. Walk with the trans community and show your support in active ways.

Centring Trans Joy also means celebrating the richness of trans and non-binary culture and creative expression. There are enormous numbers of trans creatives. Appreciate these:

- *It's Raining Them* by Mila Jam.
    www.youtube.com/watch?v=H285MJRP_Mo
- *Home* by Michaela Jae Rodriguez.
    www.youtube.com/watch?v=NkLEFzOHnEY
- *Love's in Need of Love* from POSE.
    www.youtube.com/watch?v=ZW-9zxW-XZc
- *Fox & Owl Fisher: Non-Binary Trans Debate.*
    www.youtube.com/watch?v=4cRBUHGpHpY
- *VISIBLE* documentary trailer by Campbell X produced by Kayza Rose.
    www.youtube.com/watch?v=38lRn2jFMj4
- Sabah Choudrey on Gender Diversity.
    www.youtube.com/watch?v=2sacaISqE4g

15 AUTHOR DIALOGUE 'THE PEARL IN THE OYSTER'

Matthew: I was recently very fortunate to have a dialogue with Sabah Choudrey, author of 'Supporting Trans People of

Colour', about resilience. Sabah is a non-binary person of colour, and they were exploring with me the idea that there is a kind of intersectionality about resilience because it will look different for each person based on the social privilege they experienced and the opportunity that gave to develop resilience, to come to know it as a skill and force within. So, from that, can I ask you, Natasha, what does resilience mean to you, and how does resilience show up for you?

Natasha: I think the definition of resilience for me is the ability to sustain discomfort – uncomfortable feelings, the ability to relate to and be with uncomfortable feelings *and* be able to hold your authentic course in life. The resilience in the eyes of dysphoria, for example – and dysphoria can be generated externally and socially of course, due to lack of acceptance, lack of understanding, and sometimes due to total ignorance. So, that creates the difficult feelings that queer and gender diverse people have to sit with, have to sustain in order to exist. We have to sustain those feelings by which I mean experience those difficult feelings and bounce back from them, we cannot be overwhelmed or broken by these feelings, otherwise we end up acting out in some form or another – using drugs, alcohol, so that we do *not* feel – essentially killing ourselves in some form.

Matthew: So, you have to exist and be with these difficulties and challenges and discomfort and not deny them, but keep moving forward with them.

Natasha: Yes, that's it. Resilience is the ability to exist and thrive even at the same time as feeling the discomfort.

Matthew: The life friction, the process of our desire to be authentic rubbing against those existential and daily challenges to being myself, and to keep going, keep bouncing back and finding those tiny victories and alternative, creative ways to be. It's the ultimate 'and, and' way of being which is that you don't deny – you know it, and you continue: I feel the discomfort and I have the resources in me to keep going.

Natasha: Yes, we are all in the process of making those pearls in the oyster, the friction that creates the pearl. Developing resilience in ourselves and our clients is about placing the emphasis on how we re-charge our batteries and make social connections, create communities of belonging, as you have said, Matthew. I would like to conclude this section by asking our readers to take time right now and think about resilience in their lives. Here are some questions:
- What does resilience look like for you?
- How have you developed your skills and capacity to respond in times of stress?
- What victories and alternative ways of being, and connections to support have you discovered in times of crisis?
- What place does solidarity have in your life?

Chapter 4

THE ADVOCATE BRIDGE

> **OVERVIEW**
> - This chapter aims to outline the core concepts of allyship, advocacy, activism, accomplice relationship, solidarity, ask etiquette, pronouns.
> - It contains Key Points 16–19.

16 LIFE COMMITMENT

Speech and language therapists lead extremely busy work lives, with large, often complex caseloads in many specialist areas. There is often little time for training and study. However, working with trans and non-binary people is not only a unique opportunity to understand potentially new cultural practices, but it facilitates deep self-learning and personal growth in the pursuit of dynamic cultural humility (Mills & Pert, 2024). Because of the historic schism between the trans community and gender services, there is a very great need to build bridges of trust and advocacy. The culture wars and transphobic outpourings in our current societal perceptions and ideology means that we must ensure that the quality of our care and advocacy going forward is of the highest standard. This might be realised simply by listening to clients and honouring their voices and stories with the space and respect they deserve. It might involve becoming active in campaigns such as banning conversion practices, promoting trans awareness within our trusts and organisations, and not being a bystander when we witness acts or words that discount, ridicule, attack or express blatant transphobia towards gender diverse people. Being a trans ally is an *emergent* status granted to us by the trans community. Review your understanding of the following roles:

- **Ally** – someone not from the marginalised group but who stands with members of that group and expresses support in attitude and behaviour every day.
- **Advocate** – someone who uses their professional and social privilege to meet challenges on behalf of the marginalised group member to ensure their needs and rights are known and met.
- **Activist** – someone who protests through direct action against the social injustice and inequality experienced and visited on the marginalised group; it is a specific kind of advocacy.
- **Accomplice** – someone not from the marginalised group but who puts themselves in the direct firing line of attack to shield the marginalised individual from the risk they are always taking.

Working with specific marginalised populations with different access needs – such as people who stammer, trans and non-binary people, Deaf people, Blind people – particularly if the field is highly politicised, as with trans culture, requires awareness of the wider power dynamics and social discourse. This means when we turn off the lights in our therapy room at the close of the working day, we keep alight and alive the principles we have reflected on and stand for in the *whole of our life* so that we remain *response-able* in any circumstance of transphobia that we meet in our life. This is what it means to have integrity and take responsibility.

> To be completely honest, I'll be quite blunt. I don't think it's possible to do your best work if you disengage from a wider setting and demonstrate empathy only in your job and not outside work. If you are not addressing how to be inclusive in all areas of your life, then I don't think

it's possible to do your best work. And I think that will always be felt by your service users.

(Zainabb Hull in Mills & Pert, 2024, p. 46)

17 WHY PRONOUNS?

Ask etiquette (Richards & Barker, 2013) is a common practice within the trans community and beyond, and is welcomed so long as the question comes with straightforward respect and genuineness: 'Can I check which pronouns you use?' We need to avoid digging into aspects of the client's life not pertinent to our professional jurisdiction, and positioning the client as our trans awareness trainer or educator. It is also important to avoid referring to the birth assignation unless there is wider multidisciplinary discussion about hormone or surgical interventions in which it may be pertinent. In voice therapy, we do not need to know a client's gender identity and birth assignation; requesting client pronouns is information enough to be effective and informed in our work. If instances arise when we need to check an aspect of a client's identity or journey, we do so sensitively. Asking for pronouns, eliciting goals and listening to the client's voice are the key components of need-to-know and of working collaboratively. It is important to steer away from the use of qualifiers such as 'prefer' or 'preference' ('her preferred name is' – no); names and pronouns are straightforwardly what people use even if the name change is not official/deed poll attained ('her name is' – yes); preference implies whimsy, and facile choice making, as though the identity expressed is not serious or valid, but trivial and insubstantial.

Stating our pronouns communicates that:

1. I am not going to make assumptions about cisness and transness being identifiable from physical appearance.
2. I am normalising the practice of giving pronouns, as a visible act of solidarity *with* and being an accomplice *for* the trans community (if I am a cis person).
3. I centre an ask etiquette culture of respect.

It is appropriate for cis people to state their pronouns before asking the same of gender diverse people, due to relative marginalisation and social risk. Many binary trans people do not initiate offering pronouns, and may feel bemused or offended when asked. This comes from an aspiration to be gendered accurately without question, which is the position most cis people expect for themselves. It takes practice to use pronouns and neopronouns (such as 'ze, zir, zirs'; 'ey, em, eir'; 'per, per, pers' [subject, object, possessive]) accurately in social contexts due to the inaugural linguistic challenge. Shlasko (2017) has developed extremely useful exercises and resources to flex our 'pronounaround' muscles.

Simply, if we slip up or make a mistake, follow these steps:

1. Say sorry.
2. Correct the mistake with a repetition using the right pronoun.
3. Move on and carry on with the conversation.

Here is an example conversation:

A: 'Did you ask if he can come?'
B: 'Erm, *they*, it is *they* … '
A: 'Sorry, did you ask if *they* can come? I think they want to join us for coffee.'

In our own time, away from the conversation and slip-up, we can quietly reflect on what may have caused the error and what we need to do *and practise* to reduce the possibility of it happening again. It is important that at the time of the mishap, we do not make a big apology or dance of guilt before the misgendered person, as this requires them both to cope with the misgendering and provide reassurance and forgiveness, placing our difficult feelings at the centre rather than those of the trans person, and our need to be rescued over what is effectively their double erasure. In particular, watch out when we are speaking in groups and potentially rushing and not giving ourselves enough time to 'plan ahead' linguistically. Also, be careful if we know someone's gender history before transition and we speak on autopilot and invoke someone as their 'former' self.

18 ACTIONS TOWARDS ALLYSHIP

Being a trans ally is not an identity cis people can claim for themselves. It is, as we have said above, an emergent position gifted to us by the trans community through our actions. Community wisdom speaks:

> I think people want to be a trans ally, to claim allyship, so that they can essentially stop doing that allyship work, so that there's an end point to learning, and they can say 'thankfully, I don't need to do anything anymore.' And that's just not the reality of the world.
> *(Zainabb Hull in Mills & Pert, 2024, pp. 75–76)*

These are actions for all people, and especially cis people, to engage and move forward with:

- Aim to be an advocate in the first instance through your actions.
- Become an activist and accomplice in difficult times – take the hit for community.
- Centre trans rights in all your work and life.
- Meet trans people where they are without assumption or judgment.
- Centre gender euphoria and Trans Joy.
- Practise pronouns in linguistic scenarios with yourself in preparation for social context.
- Pronoun yourself in your email addresses, Zoom profile names, Teams profiles, conversations which feel doable; ask your colleagues and friends if they can do the same.
- When making a mistake: apologise, correct the error, move on.

- Review and use language which includes and creates belonging.
- Notice hierarchy and othering and find alternatives which create commonality.
- Do the work on yourself, develop positionality and challenge yours and other people's.
- Place lived experience at the centre of your work – be co-productive in your therapy.
- Create spaces which are confidential, welcoming and sensitive to intersectional identities.
- Actively challenge transphobia and discrimination whenever you hear it – do not stand by, do not amplify myths by remaining silent in the face of prejudice.
- Learn about, learn from and celebrate trans culture and trans creative people.
- Know the colours of the trans flag (white, light blue, pink) and the non-binary flag (yellow, white, purple and black).

19 AUTHOR DIALOGUE 'WALKING WITH AND TAKING THE HIT'

Matthew: Thanks for your wisdom and perspective about theory and practice and action above, Natasha.

Natasha: Well, this book aims to be succinct and useful, we hope.

Matthew: So, Natasha, can I ask you specifically what 'ally' means to you?

Natasha: Yes, an 'ally' for me is aiming to be a positive, supportive, boundaried friend. An ally is a friend in some sense because they demonstrate empathy for the struggle even if they are not fully in the struggle themselves. And there is the important concept of 'showing up' – of being there. An ally shows up and walks with those of us who struggle. They take a hit from normative attack, they stand with us in solidarity against gender critical ideology, they stand trans-affirmatively tall and firm in the face of culture wars and oppositional hate politics.

Matthew: And we are growing into being an ally.

Natasha: Yes, don't aim to be an ally, aim to be affirmative of trans people, an advocate, an activist. Please don't let words of discrimination and hate pass you by. Don't ask people their gender identity – just pronoun yourself and politely ask someone for their pronouns if the context requires and if you are in an individual setting. Trans people are diverse, ordinary, extraordinary, kind, caring, hurting, struggling, surviving, trying, hoping, crying, and loving and deserve as much respect as any human being.

Matthew: We are humans together in the circle of all life concern.

Natasha: Solidarity, yes – we look forward to a future of peace, of hope, of diversity and aspiration. We have it today.

Matthew: It heralds a new future.

Natasha: Absolutely. Hope is not nebulous.

Matthew: I like the story told by a Buddhist monk who when asked 'is your cup of life half full or half empty?', replied, 'I am grateful that I have a cup.'

Natasha: That's beautiful.

Chapter 5

OVERVIEW OF GENDER-AFFIRMING MEDICAL INTERVENTIONS

> **OVERVIEW**
> - This chapter aims to outline the core concepts of hormone replacement therapy, surgeries related to medical transition, Three 'A's Principles, voyeurism.
> - It contains Key Points 20–21.

20 HORMONES AND SURGERIES

In the recent past, training courses and orientation lectures in trans healthcare were fashioned to include in-depth surgical and endocrinological information, diagrams and pictures. This has attracted warranted criticism from the trans community as being potentially voyeuristic. Clearly, looking at pre- and post-surgical pictures of genital reconstructions needs very sensitive handling. Surgeon and endocrinologist colleagues now specifically tailor the instruction and training for allied health professionals so we emerge as sensitively informed and collaborative members of the gender service multidisciplinary team which prioritises the autonomy, privacy and safety of our clients. Speech and language therapists need to have an overview of hormone and surgery interventions so that we understand in adequate terms what clients may be going through and we can make appropriate adjustments and adaptations to voice therapy, and the appointment timing/scheduling while clients are, for example, preparing for gamete storage, commencing hormone therapy, or recovering from surgery. We are informed by the careful approaches of Dr Kate Nambiar, Endocrinology Specialist for the Welsh Gender Service, and Miss Tina Rashid, Consultant Urologist and NHS England Clinical Lead for Surgery (Gender Dysphoria). Nambiar advocates the *Three 'A's Principles* – authenticity, autonomy, accessibility (Mills & Pert, 2024). Authenticity means trans and non-binary people achieve the physical changes and body authentic to them, irrespective of what is socially or normatively 'expected.' Autonomy means that trans and non-binary people are in charge of what is happening in and with their body. Accessibility means centring an open access, co-productive and supportive client-clinician relationship and dialogue where trans and non-binary people are not assessed related to a model of pathology, but where clients have access to the advice, treatment and support they require. Remember that the system of assessing clients for and diagnosing them with *Gender Incongruence* facilitates trans people's access to treatment. Diagnosis must never be used as a justification not to treat people. Also, note that there used to be an accepted protocol within speech and language therapy that the client could not be seen unless they had stepped into living full-time in their affirmed gender role, and were under a gender service. Today, the service specifications are more inclusive. Speech and language therapists see any gender diverse client – women, men, non-binary people – those who have not changed names, those who have; those who have not made a full-time social transition but are transitioning in a more personal way. We may very well see gender diverse clients in speech and language therapy not related to care in transition, but to broader life healthcare after transition where the trans and cis person, though needing slight adaptations to certain procedures and access to others, are simply part of the general population. Tables 5.1, 5.2 and 5.3 provide an overview of changes produced by hormone replacement therapy and surgeries related to medical transition. For more information, look at Vincent (2018, 2020).

Table 5.1 Testosterone HRT

Hormone Replacement Therapy Oriented to trans men, transmasculine people, non-binary transmasculine people	
Testosterone (commonly referred to as 't')	
Administration	Injectable, patches, pumps
Secondary sex changes	<ul><li>Increased body hair.</li><li>Increased facial hair.</li><li>Increase muscle mass.</li><li>Increased thickening of skin.</li><li>Vocal fold thickening (some slight increases to laryngeal cartilage) – usually commences after 3–4 months on t, usually finishes growth at 12–18 months (injectable sustanon [monthly] or nebido [three-monthly] faster acting and effects take longer to cease than topical gels via pumps and patches).</li><li>Increased libido.</li><li>Increased appetite.</li><li>Increased emotional volatility.</li><li>Hair loss.</li><li>Menstruation cessation.</li><li>Clitoral growth.</li></ul>

Table 5.2 Oestrogen and Testosterone Blockers HRT

Hormone Replacement Therapy Oriented to trans women, transfeminine people, non-binary transfeminine people	
Oestrogen	
Administration	Tablets, patches, pumps
Secondary sex changes	<ul><li>Reduced body hair.</li><li>Reduced facial hair.</li><li>Breast development.</li><li>Fat redistribution.</li><li>Reduction and cessation in erectile function.</li><li>Genitalia atrophy.</li><li>Reduction in libido.</li><li>Increased connection to emotional sensitivity and lability.</li></ul>
Testosterone blockers	
Administration	Injectables, tablets.
Effects	suppression of testosterone production.

Table 5.3 Gender-Affirming Surgeries Associated with Medical Transition

Gender-Affirming Surgeries Associated with Medical Transition	
Oriented to trans men, transmasculine people, non-binary transmasculine people	Oriented to trans women, transfeminine people, non-binary transfeminine people
<ul><li>Hysterectomy.</li><li>Bilateral salpingo-oophorectomy (removal of fallopian tubes and ovaries).</li><li>Double mastectomy and masculine/neutral chest reconstruction (often referred to as 'top surgery').</li><li>Metoidioplasty (formation of phallus from clitoris).</li><li>Phalloplasty (creation of phallus from arm or leg skin graft).</li><li>Facial masculinisation.</li><li>Phonosurgery (type III thyroplasty).</li></ul>	<ul><li>Vulvoplasty (creation of vulva without a vaginal cavity).</li><li>Vaginoplasty (creation of vulva and vagina with cavity, requiring dilation maintenance) – often referred to as GRS meaning 'genital reconstruction surgery' **not** 'gender reassignment surgery' [surgery does not reassign gender, it aligns the body with someone's felt sense of gender].</li><li>Penectomy (removal of penis).</li><li>Bilateral orchidectomy (removal of testes).</li><li>Thyroid chondroplasty (reduction in thyroid notch) – sometimes referred to as 'tracheal shave' – is a cosmetic procedure which does not affect the voice, unless the reduction is too great and detaches the vocal folds which is a serious circumstance for the voice).</li><li>Phonosurgery (cricothyroid approximation, glottoplasty, vocal fold muscle reduction) – largely aimed to raise pitch; some changes reported to resonance experience; limitations to singing voice; surgical risks of dysphonia and globus pharygeus.</li><li>Facial feminisation.</li></ul>

21 AUTHOR DIALOGUE 'PLEASE LISTEN TO ME'

Matthew: So, thinking about the importance of hormones, what has been significant for you in your journey with hormones, Natasha?

Natasha: When I started my gender transition, my medical transition was an important part of it, as was my social transition. And a big part of many medical gender transitions is HRT, or hormone replacement therapy, which happens at sex hormones level. I was prescribed those through the NHS, and it felt like it was a long time coming, as I was expecting them to come a bit earlier. It took a couple of years from when I was referred to the gender clinic before I was able to access hormone replacement. But once I did, they impacted a lot and very positively on my journey.

Matthew: Could you say something about the terminology 'hormone replacement therapy,' Natasha?

Natasha: Yes, personally, the term stems from that I was living in a body that was recognised as male, and that body had a lot of testosterone running through it and not much oestrogen. Therefore, the *replacement* is of the sex hormones and adding to the oestrogen, which is a typically female hormone, while reducing the testosterone – a typically male hormone – and finding a new balance in the body that actually *feels more congruent and better.*

Matthew: Thanks for your lived expertise and insight. Terms like 'feminising' hormones are around, but how do we ensure we are not erasing people with non-binary identities with our terms?

Natasha: Better to say simply hormone replacement therapy (HRT). There is a huge range of changes and effects people want to achieve – trans women, trans men, non-binary people, gender fluid people, bi-gender people. As I have stated, I identify as a binary trans woman, and therefore wanted to *feminise* my body as much as I could, starting from the deficit of inhabiting a typically male body. And it took a few years actually before the hormones produced visible results, like the development of female secondary sex characteristics – smoother skin, less body hair and breast growth etc., were all significant changes, and hormone replacement enabled these changes to happen. And, yes, there are people who are happy with a mix of physical characteristics and take bespoke HRT to find the balance in their bodies that feels comfortable for them. And there's no particular end point, as these can change at any point, and how we treat our bodies, the hormones that we take can change, as well as how we want to present and how we want to feel. Many people may experience gender as being dynamic, and so a transition of gender should be dynamic too.

Matthew: That's really important, because I would imagine many readers will have a sense that it's a process of starting hormones, then development, then it's all done and then you go on living. Many people take low dose hormones and then maybe stop and start again, or change administration – some trans men start t via topical gel and then when they feel more confident they move to t given in injectable form. This can often be the case with singers who want to progress slowly with the vocal change, though there are pros and cons with that.

Natasha: You are right. It's about what makes one feel comfortable, finding a personal balance in themselves. Hormones play a huge part in how we feel and how we sense our bodies to be.

Matthew: Where does fertility preservation fit into the journey?

Natasha: With regards to preservation of fertility, I personally had my sperm frozen about ten years ago when I started HRT, and it's still in a freezer somewhere in London waiting for it to either be used or thrown away – whichever I decide. There are options for people to have their DNA frozen in order for them to preserve the chances of having their own biological children in the future if they want to, and that's something that needs to be done before you start HRT, although one might be able to stop it for a while and resume being fertile – so it's not 'black and white.'

Matthew: This is a bit controversial – the idea that for cis people who don't experience incongruence with their body, there might be a sense that body change, body transformation through hormones or surgeries or both is akin to harming the body. I wonder whether you can give your thoughts about the importance of bodily autonomy?

Natasha: Certainly. I say, with respect to the readers – please listen to me. The body autonomy of the trans person is central, totally central. The ability to modify and alter my body, through hormone replacement therapy and surgical interventions has been an essential part of my personal experience of being a trans person. Without the ability that comes through medicine, medication and surgeries included, I would not be able to live a balanced life as I wanted it to be. I feel like it is indeed *my right* to change my body in ways that feel comfortable, and give me congruence and balance in myself. And I can finally see myself the way that I want to see myself. And I say finally, although there is not necessarily an endpoint to this. But at some point, I want to be able to have balance in myself and my body, and that happened for me through body modification. And, of course, there are risks involved in interventions, like a raised risk of cancer through HRT, or the risk of surgeries going wrong in some way. But at the same time, when we don't look from a cis-centric perspective, we understand that there is a need for that. So, these associated risks are *calculated* risks, not just unthought out, haphazard or whimsical things that we do to our bodies. No, they are things we do in order to achieve balance and congruence and happiness.

Matthew: Thank you for your frankness, Natasha. Can we discuss the thorny (for some) topic of puberty blockers? There was a very public court case in the UK recently which sought to stop or limit adolescent trans people taking puberty blockers, and then the High Court actually overturned that decision, wisely. There has been a great deal of erroneous and harmful press coverage.

Natasha: Yes, young and adolescent trans people were being formulated as not as competent in and about ourselves as young and adolescent cis people and the High Court rightly overturned a transphobic judgment. And for me, puberty blockers can be life-saving, and I am mean to use a very strong language here. I stress *life-saving* because, and I will speak of myself, if I had been able to avoid going through the wrong type of puberty in my adolescence, I would have saved myself from a great deal of mental-health anguish and subsequent damage. The fact that there are medications in use, recommended by international experts in the field, that enable young people to avoid going through the undesirable effects of the wrong puberty, can be absolutely life-saving. I think puberty suppressants give time for a young person to think about their gender carefully and to think about how they want to approach their future, giving them an opportunity to mould themselves in a much more efficient way, and of course this is done gently and compassionately with trans affirmative clinicians and with the support and love of family members. Because when you go through puberty as I did, I witnessed my skeletal structure grow in ways that I didn't want it – my hands grew, my head grew, my face changed, and it was all really, really traumatic. I went through a horribly traumatic experience through puberty, knowing from a young age that I wasn't male, and still going through a male puberty. And to be able to avoid or delay or reduce that type of traumatic experience with the help of certain types of medications, I believe is indeed life-affirming.

Matthew: This is very moving, Natasha. We benefit from you being so articulate about your own challenges and process, the resilience, compassion you have developed and insight you impart. I think our readers will have your expert account resounding in their ears, and take your words deeply to heart. Thank you.

Chapter 6

FUNDAMENTAL PRINCIPLES OF GENDER-AFFIRMING VOICE EXPLORATION

> **OVERVIEW**
> - This chapter aims to outline the core concepts journeying, authenticity, plurality, code switching, collaboration, relational voice, pedagogy, conscious competence, imposter syndrome.
> - It contains Key Points 22–28.

22 VOCAL JOURNEYING

There are fundamental principles which underpin and guide you to gender-affirming voice exploration. They arise from the intersections of trans cultural humility, effective voice coaching and therapeutic skill, and serve as a measure of the quality of your collaboration with your clients. Understanding their significance and absorbing them into the *essence* of your practice, means you have the intention to embody and develop really useful and accountable voice therapy, mindfully positioned and tuned to the trans person you are working with and whom you serve (Figure 6.1).

Trans and non-binary people do not have a voice disorder. This is one of the most important sentences of this book. Rehabilitation of a voice *problem* of behavioural or organic aetiology rests on the principle of returning a voice (where

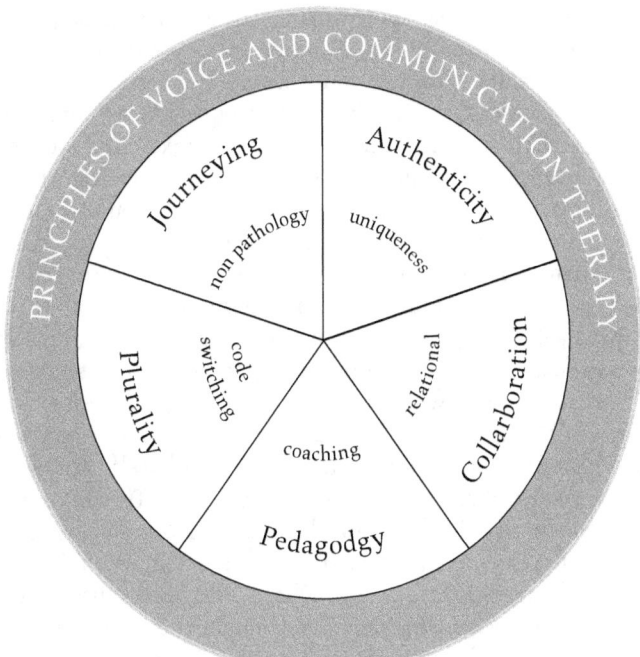

Figure 6.1 Fundamental Principles Underpinning Trans Voicing Exploration

possible) to a state of health and function previously known, alongside enabling the client to understand the causal factors and be psychologically resolved. In voice exploration with trans and non-binary people, we move from medicalising terminology which centres pathology to the nomenclature of therapy, pedagogy and vocal journeying. To understand and acknowledge both the history of pathologisation and the current wide-scale dehumanisation of trans people, as discussed in Chapter 3, means that using disorder-oriented nomenclature in the context of gender-affirming voice exploration is to continue the very real harm done to our clients. Therefore, we have: not assessment but initial appointment; not diagnostics pinpointing disease but expansion and enjoyment of vocal identity and performance; not treatment but therapy and coaching; not an outcome predicated on return but outcomes about client congruence charting multi-skills in multi-contexts on a journey of discovery; not adjunctive techniques but vocal *technique* and impact in constant development towards conscious and unconscious competence; not deference to clinical expertise, but collaborative and co-productive alliance of lived and clinical experience with multidirectional learning.

Michael White, innovator of Narrative Therapy, drew on Van Gennep's 'Rites of Passage' metaphor to describe a *migration* of identity in which the client undertakes a desired but potentially fraught and discombobulating yet surprising journey towards living more authentically with self-care, self-compassion and self-awareness (White, 2007). The migration of vocal identity (Mills & Stoneham, 2017, 2021) and journeys of vocal development (Mills & Pert, 2024) extend White's work into landscapes of trans voicing where skills are (re)discovered, obstacles are tackled, resilience is strengthened, and support is embraced. New destinations and possibilities of voicing, communicating and being emerge from liminal spaces as vocal home, vocal comfort and vocal euphoria. Journeys may be trepidatious, even fearful, but lead to greater self-value and confidence.

23 VOCAL AUTHENTICITY

To be human is to be bodily separate yet with an intrinsic need to be seen and heard, a desire to connect, share and walk alongside our fellow beings (including our relationship with animals and plants) – not only the circle of *human* concern but that of *all life*. We experience and process ourselves from one moment to the next subjectively, intrapersonally and intuitively, and we steer our self-perception through the terrain of the perception of others.

We have an innate connection between sensing our sound through bone conduction and releasing it into the world unselfconsciously to express our needs, unencumbered by how our sound may be perceived by others. We do this until we meet the vulnerability of not being heard in a way we intended, of being judged vocally at some level and being found wanting. Recordings of our voice, however high in quality, are by definition *in* and *of the past*, and therefore we can listen back to our voice only post mortem, as it were. Therefore, it is the human solution to be true to ourselves in the first instance, to be congruent, to live according to our own directive, to connect with our right to speak, to make do and thrive within our vocal skin. No one can be and sound who we are but we, ourselves. This is vocal authenticity. This means we support our clients to acknowledge and navigate the *paradox of change* (self-expression vis a vis normative expectation) and claim conscious ownership of the intention to explore and find voice(s), codes and expressions that are the client's totally personal vocal profile and communication map (Mills & Stoneham, 2017, 2021; Mills & Pert, 2024). Agency fosters engagement, determination, playfulness and skill development vis a vis social compromise and survival towards personal euphoria.

Many trans and non-binary people seek no vocal adjustment or change. Some clients begin voice therapy with a strong direction of travel towards a desired outcome, some need to inhabit vocal possibilities before focussing, filtering and steering. There are clients who are motivated to, and achieve a vocal performance typically and straightforwardly perceived as the gender expression they intend. This takes work, and there is cost–benefit to be made transparent. Most clients wish to make subtle changes in vocal home place, and more significant changes in certain vocal codes, and continue to refine skills in the context of living life.

It is vital that the cis voice clinician does not set up (consciously or unwittingly) a cis-standard of passing and failing. As we have discussed, the term 'passing' is highly loaded and must never be used or initiated by the cis therapist due to the inherent power cis clinicians have to privilege, assume or enforce (again, even unwittingly) cisheteronormative bias. Many clients state their desired goal to 'pass' vocally in the sense that they want to blend in to the social environment without question or negative approach, and of course, it is our duty of care as therapists to support the client in this. We do so by owning our clinical privilege and making our position transparent that we do not judge the client's voice related to 'passing' but understand, facilitate and celebrate the client's vocal choices. Some clients aim to create and sustain aspects of voice within what we describe as a 'typically perceived gendered sound by the general public,' as a means to avoid or reduce the many physical and emotional threats and dangers of being seen and heard as trans in an intensely and increasingly transphobic world. We support this by developing a standpoint which aligns to the truth that every voice is totally unique, and that there are as many feminine voices as there are women, masculine voices as there are men, non-binary voices as there are non-binary people, queer voices as there are queer people, and so on.

24 VOCAL PLURALITY

We do not have one voice, or a single voicing habit or persona. Rather, it is authentic to have many voices (voicings) that emanate from our one larynx and vocal tract. We subtly shift from a familiar 'how my voice is most of the time' ('the vocal home') to different tones, expressions, weights, qualities, formalities, intimacies, in varying contexts and temporalities. We all make subtle, sometimes dramatic gear changes, at times consciously, often subconsciously, to meet the myriad of vocal possibilities and relationship demands. Code-switching can be playful and practised creatively, but it is essentially a survival strategy. In addition, there is an emerging understanding that many people identify with plural and distinctly different voices which communicate aspects of ourselves linked to various ages of psychosocial development and responses to conflict, crisis and trauma. Several psychotherapeutic approaches formulate specific representations of the self as inner child, inner critic, critical adult, compassionate self, and inner wise observer. All such aspects of self may be perceived and experienced by the individual as sounding different inside us, and we may speak them out with particular voices and characteristics. Meg-John Barker has lectured and written compassionately and wisely in this field. See www.rewriting-the-rules.com/zines/.

Mapping voice exploration to specific code switches and configurations of vocal identity enables the client to use voice skills playfully and flexibly. This 'communication mapping' loosens any pressure or expectation to produce the untruth of the fixed and homogenised 'one-voice-fits all' fallacy. When clients speak of wanting to achieve more consistency, this is related to the consistency of using specific skills in specific contexts with conscious and unconscious competence.

We raise an important note here about *imposter syndrome* related to voice work. Exploring new sounds away from the known and familiar (the current vocal home locus), invokes imposter syndrome and anxiety about being perceived as 'putting on' a voice, that by definition sounds fake, forced, insincere or inauthentic. It can be that voice therapy actually *increases* vocal gender dysphoria for a period of time at the beginning of the process until the client becomes more skilled and able to occupy conscious competence and positively claim their developing prowess in many possibilities. Hypervigilant and critical self-monitoring blocks self-compassion and is a form of internalised policing – what we describe as 'vocal self-othering.' Being in flow and trying things out playfully are the antidotes. Giving ourselves permission to be, include and integrate all aspects of our vocal identities, however extreme, fledgling and unfamiliar those textures and colours, means we connect to the core of who we are and our vocal essence. This is vocal belonging.

25 VOCAL COLLABORATION

Vocal collaboration describes how both therapy and voice work are set up by the therapist, how the voice practitioner holds the client in therapeutic contact, guides the sessions, and locates their vocal processing in relation to and in service of that of their clients. This is described as *relational voice work* (Mills &

Stoneham, 2021; Mills & Pert, 2024). Essentially the voice therapist has developed through their own voice awareness, skill and development, and knows how to facilitate and demonstrate pitch, resonance and vocal fold weight exercises and 'experiments', which *takes account of the client's* range/resonance/weight, relative to the therapist's. For example, if the therapist is unable to pitch at D3, they need to demonstrate at D4 and explain how that sits in their range and resonance in a different way to those of D3 in the client. Alternatively, the therapist demonstrates another pitch in their voice relative to the 'step up' that the client is aiming for in their own. Ultimately this collaborative process is about facilitating conscious and understandable voice change which opens up exploration and discovery rather than shuts it down leaving the client feeling they need to copy the actual voice of the therapist, rather than using it as a model and scaffold towards their own target pitch and resonance profile. If this process is not made conscious on the part of the cis therapist, the client will feel subtly and systemically cis-assessed, and shamed. This collaboration of clinical and lived expertise tracks how therapist and client are in both psychological and vocal *contact*. There is space for shared experience, which can include the therapists' discerning and healthy disclosure and acknowledgement of where they are themselves vocally, imperfections, habits and all.

26 VOCAL PEDAGOGY

As the therapist is skilled in creating and holding a safe, confidential space for the client's self-discovery, the pedagogue knows the art, practice and methodology of teaching and coaching experientially acquired skills. Vocal pedagogy is nimble, perspicacious and truthful vocal teaching practice. The vocal pedagogue is able to connect the client to their voice-within and the desired vocal filters; they can explain rationale, demonstrate a spectrum of vocal parameters, scaffold try-outs and practice, review, challenge and give on-point, constructive feedback based on deep listening and felt sense, and adapt flexibly to learning preferences and access needs. The voice coach supports the client on a trajectory which begins didactically and segues into therapist redundancy and client independence. This process is described both in the *apprenticeship* and *conscious-competence* models, that stages of which are:

- **Unconscious incompetence** (unaware of skill and has no proficiency in it): ***The Novice***.
- **Conscious incompetence** (aware of the importance of the skill but lacks proficiency): ***The Apprentice.***
- **Conscious competence** (developing proficiency and can use skills when focussing on them): ***The Journeyperson*** becoming ***The Craftsperson***.
- **Unconscious competence** (can perform skills expertly and automatically): ***The Expert/Master Craftsperson***.

We must note that voice specialist speech and language therapists (voice therapists for short) are not voice coaches in isolation. The journey of acquisition to mastery of skills takes place within a person-centred therapeutic process. This means trans voicing exploration occurs within therapy that supports the whole person to experience and face sensitivity, vocal gender dysphoria, imposter syndrome, self-doubt, anxiety, shame; to discover competence, playfulness and new stories; and to develop intersectional resilience, agency and self-care towards vocal victories and euphoria. In effect, voice therapy blends both the being of therapy and the doing of coaching. Coaching of course centres motor learning, where praxis and repetition are core to the work. We need to be precise and motivational in helping clients towards their goals, yet sensitive to the shifts and arrivals in destination the client discovers and embraces. This is 'doing the work and letting go' (Mills & Pert, 2024). We need to develop our skills in vocal masking, rhythmic and structured turn-taking and counting in, in using biofeedback (especially visual and kinaesthetic approaches – which the abstraction of voice work requires in order to make the work more concrete, understandable and repeatable). Outcomes are valid when they capture the dynamic and congruent journey as storied by the client. Simplistic 'before' and 'after' outcomes which centre the therapist in the absence of the richness of the client narrative may subtly invite the audience/witness into a cis-assessment of the client, which you will have well understood by now is invalidating and entirely not what this work is about.

27 THERAPEUTIC AFFIRMATIONS

We offer the following *affirmations* to guide you in your voice and communication therapy practice. Affirmations are mantras or statements of intent that you can speak out openly to your clients, and/or have and hold as your therapeutic aspirations and goals for your developing and ever-refining competence.

- **Vocal Journeying**: I will accompany and support you through a landscape of familiar and new possibilities towards your vocal comfort and euphoria.
- **Vocal Authenticity**: I am in service of you to find and celebrate your authentic voice and voices, knowing fully that every voice is unique, and that there are as many feminine voices as there are women, masculine voices as there are men, and non-binary voices as there are non-binary people.
- **Vocal Plurality**: I will help you to discover and embrace connection, flow and belonging in all your voices and code switches according to the multi-contexts of your life.
- **Vocal Collaboration**: I will use my voice and voice skills relationally with you to scaffold your discovery of and enjoyment in your vocal skill and prowess.
- **Vocal Pedagogy**: I will coach you towards your vocal independence and my redundancy and celebrate your arrival and onward vocal journeys.

28 AUTHOR DIALOGUE 'TRANS VOICING'

Matthew: So, in this dialogue, I would like to ask you about a number of terms and concepts we have raised in the topics, and expand on these together now.
Natasha: Yes, of course, drill in to the details.

Matthew: So, you have spoken before, Natasha, about 'trans voicing.' This seems like a cornerstone concept for trainee speech and language therapists and newly qualified therapists to get their heads around and take to heart. What does 'trans voicing' mean to you and how might it be different to simply 'trans voice'?

Natasha: Trans voicing is all-encompassing, because it's voicing that can be seen and heard as temporal. It's not static. It's something that moves, changes, evolves, that expands, that diminishes – it doesn't matter what direction it takes, but it can take many directions, many journeys, and destinations on a continual journey which in some ways has no end point.

Matthew: It's something dynamic.

Natasha: Yes, dynamic. It's a gerund – voicing – it's a process.

Matthew: A becoming – it's more than a stock phrase, it becomes a therapist affirmation to say to a client that 'every day is a new day with your voice.' And, Natasha, is there a 'cis voicing'? I mean, do you think that there are trans and cis voices? Are these categories helpful or not?

Natasha: I would say that if we were to separate trans and cis voices, we would be drawing upon the old-school standard of separation between trans and cis, and gender as a rigid binary and gender as reductive, as gender can be perceived in society. But if we were to look at a creative present and a future which honours all of us, there would not be a separation imposed or conceptualised between trans and cis voices, because voices are on a range, definitely on a spectrum, any voice comes as part of a greater spectrum of sound, and that spectrum doesn't have to be any gender specific.

Matthew: That's brilliant, Natasha. And very helpful, because it is existentially and practically true. So, onto another point of language. We have also discussed the difference between 'techniques' and 'vocal technique.'

Natasha: Yes – a subtle but important difference.

Matthew: Voice is a whole entity. Yes, we can have strategies to survive in that moment, and thrive in others. On the phone, for example, where there's no visual cue, I can do certain things with my voice definitely, consciously, script practised, that get me through. I like to say skills rather than techniques because 'techniques' feels a little reductive or making something like 'the icing on the cake' and we need to have an *overall technique* which involves many skills – and this is akin to delving into the depth of the cake!

Natasha: Yes, it's about using language which really values the work and the person. 'Techniques' – plural – sounds like periphery work or cursory engagement, whereas 'skills' sounds like someone is really taking time to discover and enjoy their vocal possibilities and potential – it's more honouring, and not discounting. I like the concept of developing vocal technique as a statement of craft – like a professional voice user – they have technique – and this, without sounding grandiose or pompous, is something we who explore voice and communication aim to develop.

Matthew: Yes, for me, it signals that we take our voice work seriously and we are moving through the stages of conscious competence, and another way to describe it is the apprenticeship model – the phases of systems mastery: from the novice, apprentice, journeyperson, craftsperson, to the expert/master craftsperson.

Natasha: I love the apprenticeship model – we can all be our own experts and find expertise, mastery, prowess, advanced skill.

Matthew: Lastly, I want to touch in on another term which needs constant pulling apart. We have written about this earlier, but I wonder what you can offer from your personal lived experience, Natasha, of the term 'passing.' Personally, I believe that a cis or cis-liminal person must not initiate the words 'passing' or 'to pass', because these are words of power that in the cis mouth judges a trans person by a cis measure. I must, though, acknowledge and help my clients achieve a sound which enables them to move through situations where they can be more typically perceived as having the gendered sound that fits with their identity – and some clients will describe this as wanting to pass and others will describe it differently. What do you think?

Natasha: Yes, that's right, Matthew, and it is one of those fundamental points that new speech and language therapists, students – even established clinicians – must consciously take on board. We have to understand our positionality in relation to what 'passing' truly means in a socio-political power structure and therefore it will have a different weight and a different bias depending whose lips utters the term. So, beware please! Of course, we have to be careful with language, how we phrase things. And 'passing', as you say, Matthew, is a very loaded word and it reaches back into many struggles historically. Language is often symbolic of something else. I would say it is important not to idealise 'passing' or idealise cisnormative society as the ideal, but to portray it as a possibility that someone can exist in that. Support your clients to make choices which are consciously examined, without judgment or rescue or unacknowledged therapist bias.

Matthew: That's really helpful, thanks for articulating this so clearly.

Natasha: Personally, I reflect and can say that as a relatively 'passing' trans woman, my problems do not stop there. Society is harsh even with people who do pass. Of course, it's a lot harder for people who don't pass because of systemic ('cis-temic') transphobia, but even if you do pass your problems do not stop there and become more in different areas. So, 'passing' must be seen as a means to an end in certain contexts, I think. As a trans person I offer this from my lived experience. But to bring this to a close – embrace the dynamic process of trans voicing – *voicing*. Let's all begin to move past the confines of vocal gender binary performance and identity – surely human voicing is so much bigger – and full of possibility.

Chapter 7

THE THERAPEUTIC JOURNEY AND RELATIONSHIP

> **OVERVIEW**
> - This chapter aims to outline the core concepts of empathy, unconditional positive regard, respect, congruence, therapeutic field, therapeutic contract, transference, countertransference, The Drama Triangle, persecutor, victim, rescuer, challenger, co-creator, facilitator.
> - It contains Key Points 29–31.

29 SKILLS AND CONDITIONS

We are not only voice coaches, we are therapists. We coach voice within a therapy 'room,' which is both physical (including digital) and energetic. We set up the therapeutic contract of confidentiality, safe-guarding and co-sharing and there is a *field of influence* between client and therapist which is about being in *psychological contact* (Mills & Stoneham, 2021). This means that everything that is within us, we the therapists – our psychological identity, vulnerability, resilience, history, life experience and self-processing – is 'in the room.' As therapists, we need to be totally aware where we 'begin and end' so that we know the difference between our psychological material and that of the client – for just as everything within us is 'in the room,' everything within the client is also 'in the room.' Ideally, we become psychologically minded through our own lived experience of being in personal growth or crisis

DOI: 10.4324/9781003299158-8

counselling or psychotherapy, and counselling skills training and personal development group work. We are in the boat together, casting off together, journeying together.

Lack of personal psychological mindedness leads to unawareness of client transference and therapist potential countertransference of uncomfortable emotions. When left unconscious, such difficult feelings can be triggered in and leak out of the therapist, creating therapeutic entanglement. In vocal terms, we have to watch when clients transfer feelings that our voice is the goal, rather than the skill we demonstrate, and be aware of our own countertransference of superiority and cis-privilege (if we are cis) (Mills & Pert, 2024).

We avoid therapist-client enmeshment by developing Rogerian *core conditions* and *counselling skills*. Carl Rogers pioneered the 'person-centred approach' which affirms that people have innate resources for self-understanding and personal growth, that clients are the experts in themselves, that therapists demonstrate trust that clients know what they need, and that the therapeutic alliance is helping and reparative in and of itself, because it centres a trusting, boundaried, human relationship where process can take place. The best thing we can do is to listen actively, so clients feel heard, seen and valued. If in doubt, simply listen. Do not jump in and try to fix; trust pause and silence. Simply, be.

Counselling skills include listening, attending, paraphrasing, summarising, asking questions, encouraging specificity, reflecting feelings, challenging when needed, enabling clarification. The core conditions embody the therapist's ideal relationship and attitude to the client (Rogers, 2004).

- **Empathy** – an ability to understand sensitively and accurately what the client is experiencing in the here and now, to follow what they are feeling and communicate that back to them.
- **Congruence** – an ability to be genuine, open and truthful, where the therapist's inside matches their outside, where the therapist is open to their own feelings and responses

and able to challenge the client when noticing ambivalence or inconsistency.
- **Unconditional Positive Regard** – the ability to express non-judgemental acceptance of the client's worth as a human being, to have genuine care of them; this can be challenging for clients raised and living under 'oppressive conditions of worth' where acceptance has been conditional and self-compassion is not easily accessible (James & Brumfitt, 2018).

As with the process of becoming a voice pedagogue, it takes time to become a sensitive and skilled therapist. There is a necessity to go beyond the brief introduction to counselling skills in our professional registration degrees, and enroll in short courses in Further Education colleges – for example, The City Literary Institute and Mary Ward Centre, London. Later in your development, you may want to pursue approaches which complement voice change and identity exploration – Mindfulness (Kabat-Zinn, 2016), Compassion Focused Therapy (Gilbert, 2015), Solution-Focused Brief Therapy (de Shazer, 2012), Narrative Therapy (White, 2007; Denborough, 2014). Use Figure 7.1 to locate and review your progress.

30 KNOW THE DRAMA

In addition to counselling skills and core conditions, there is a psychological model from Transactional Analysis (Berne, 2010) that we find absolutely invaluable. Observing the mechanisms of The Drama Triangle (Karpman, 1968) both in your human interactions and in your work as a therapist will change your life. The Drama Triangle describes three unprocessed, dysfunctional human relationships (roles/positions) between two or more people that we all adopt in times of social stress and threat. They are coping strategies formed in early childhood, the operation of each role/position being largely unconscious as we flit from one to another in rapid succession. We may favour one or two roles/positions, but the ultimate outcome is that everyone remains in *victim*. Not until we become conscious of how each role/position is activated within us and shapes our

THE THERAPEUTIC JOURNEY AND RELATIONSHIP

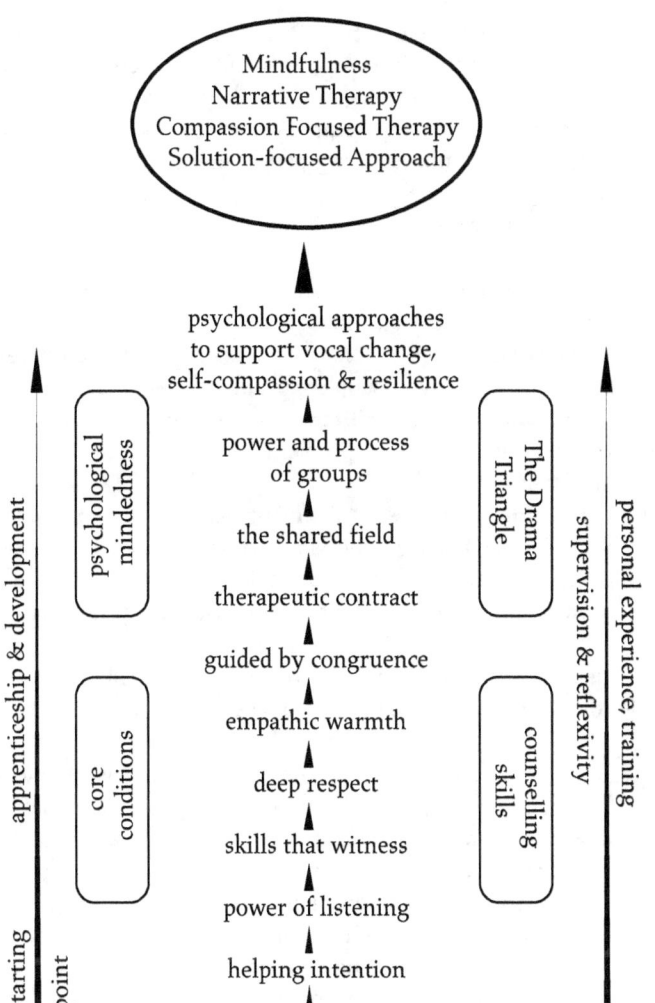

Figure 7.1 In Psychological Contact within Voice Therapy

interactions, are we able to transform ours and another's role/position, thereby enabling empowerment, not victimhood, for all. The three roles/positions and how they express themselves are below. It is important to emphasise that they are not actual life roles – we are not labelling people literally as persecutor, victim or rescuer – they are *psychological processes* bubbling up from our subconscious.

- **Victim** (expresses powerlessness, helplessness and invitation to be rescued) *becomes* **Co-creator** (who has agency, initiates committed action and can negotiate and self-care).
- **Rescuer** (takes over people's problems and makes them their own) *becomes* **Facilitator** (who supports without hurrying to solve people's problems or feeling pressured to give answers).
- **Persecutor** (expresses punishment, blame and aggression) *becomes* **Challenger** (who is assertive not aggressive, and firm and fair in resetting boundaries and reminding people of the consequences of their actions without punishment).

Let us consider three scenarios to observe how transforming the roles leads to client (and therapist) empowerment:

1. When the client arrives for the first time, they will almost certainly feel nervous. The power dynamic is weighted to the therapist. The client may evoke the therapist as the magician, healer, fixer or wand waver – and in so doing, cast themselves subconsciously as victim and invite the therapist to be their rescuer. It is important for the therapist to be welcoming and *facilitating*, where we gently hand back the archetype of the expert in the course of the therapy sessions, enabling the client to become a co-creator.
2. We become therapists likely because we are deeply motivated to make helping relationships. However, therapists need to be especially careful how our inner rescuer manifests in the therapy space – the 'oh, poor you' mechanism. If we rescue, we cast the client as victim; they

will ultimately become irritated, unconsciously, at being evoked as helpless, will be activated into anger and become 'persecutory', acting out with active or passive aggression. If we are unconscious of this process, we in turn become victim to the client's persecutor, and so it goes around. When we remain facilitator, challenger, co-creator, we invite the client to step into their power in the same way.

3. If a client has not practised vocally or does not achieve an exercise accurately or is somehow seemingly disengaged, we may express unconscious frustration, perhaps because we are having a bad day or our inner resources are squeezed due to the pressures and stressors upon us. When we behave in this way, we have stepped into persecutor and invite the client into remaining in victimhood. If we are therapists and voice coaches who are too wedded to our expertise and certainty, we are too far ahead of the client and stifle client discovery. We therapists must be humble and sacrifice the unconscious need and secondary gains of being seen as expert; when we risk being 'found out' we demonstrate our common humanity and our imperfections and we enable ourselves and the client to be co-creators, not persecutor-rescuer and victim.

When we transform our role/position, we enable our relationship in the boat to be truly collaborative, a shared journey and a shared odyssey (Mills & Pert, 2024).

31 AUTHOR DIALOGUE 'IN THE BOAT TOGETHER'

Matthew: We have spoken before about the image of being in the boat as deeply collaborative.

Natasha: Yes, it's a great image. Setting out on a journey – the therapist has the skills to be with someone, and allows their skills to develop on the journey. They go on a journey of discovery together. And therapists need to develop those counselling skills – at the core of this, it's about just being human, having empathy and employing Carl Rogers' core conditions in every minute of your work with your client.

Matthew: Being empathic.

Natasha: Yes, being fully positive in the regard that we receive clients who are trying to change, or expand or develop their voice, finding their authentic voice and voices.

Matthew: Yes, voices, as the possibility models include code switches and *plurality* of voice.

Natasha: Certainly, so. And we connect with and hold the struggle that clients have in exploring voicing, the struggles that stem almost exclusively from transphobia. And because of that transphobia, external or internalised, we need to enable clients to develop their resilience, but also remember that they are, as we are, human. And it's OK to hurt, it's OK to be in pain, it's OK the be in discomfort, it's even OK to be dysphoric at times and then what the therapist does is to be human – we receive our clients as equals and we are supportive, empathic, congruent and we do not see our clients as other, we empathise and above all listen – yes, essentially – listen to their struggle without trying to change it or telling them that they are somehow wrong in one shape or other for feeling that way.

Matthew: The power of listening.

Natasha: Yes, it's the simplest thing in some ways just to listen, but to really listen takes practice. The conundrum for the voice therapist is that you have to be voice teachers and voice therapists – so that means you have *doing* and *being* to be negotiated in the voice work. It's not psychological talking therapy, but it is voice work and a kind *vocal psychotherapy*. Rather incredible when it's done well.

Chapter 8

ORIENTATION TO GENDER-AFFIRMING VOICE AND COMMUNICATION THERAPY

> **OVERVIEW**
> - This chapter aims to outline the core concepts and practices of coaching ethics, experiential voice work, motor learning principles, practical pedagogy, more on imposter syndrome, the initial appointment, High-Bright-Thin voice work, Low-Chest-Thick voice work, non-binary voicing, client-centred journeys and outcomes.
> - It contains Key Points 32–47.

32 COACHING ETHICS

Look back at the discussion of the principles which underpin gender-affirming voice exploration (Section 7). By now, you have the statement emblazoned on your notebook that this work is not about pathology – neither of personhood, nor of vocal function and identity. Yet, here is the conundrum. The speech and language therapist specialising in voice has a professional role and post registration training to work in voice disorders within an ENT pathway. Notwithstanding intersectional experience, by contrast the voice coach is trained to work with voice in performance, education and the creative arts, and is a skilled practitioner and pedagogue, developed through a professional voice training at a conservatoire of music or drama, through training as a teacher of speech, drama and text, or as a theatre practitioner and director. How, then, can the speech and language therapist without professional voice training develop vocal pedagogical competence? Certainly, skills gained in voice therapy models and approaches – such as Estill Voice Training (Steinhauer et al., 2017), Lessac-Masden Resonant Voice Therapy (Verdolini Abbott, 2008) – are highly relevant and adaptive to voice coaching. But we need to go further: voice and communication therapy is the holistic exploration of whole voice into the unknown, which means that the therapist's voice, vocal processing and skill are *intrinsic* to the journey.

The ethics of coaching – teaching the acquisition of physical behaviours and skills towards mastery – be we a voice coach, piano teacher or driving instructor, means that we not only need to know *how* to do it, but that we need to have *made conscious our process in knowing how* to do it so that we can coach those behaviours to a novice, a trainee, a skilled and an expert practitioner and craftsperson. **We cannot teach what we do not know**. For example, you would not countenance being taught to drive by someone who cannot drive themselves but who has read a manual of theory, can describe the vehicle dimensions, parts and operations, and knows the rules of the highway code. What you need is an experienced *driver*, able to manoeuvre the car in all speeds and road contexts, who is also an experienced *instructor*.

Let your passion to become a really useful and effective therapist in this field be your motivation to gain the skills you currently lack. You can develop your voice easily through regular and focused practice, and start today. We recommend that you do the work by yourself, as well as reach out to the many voice development courses in Further Education colleges, learning opportunities in relevant Clinical Excellence Network workshops, and more substantial post graduate programmes such as the renowned MA/MFA in Voice Studies at the Royal Central School of Speech and Drama. *All we say in this key point is that you set yourself on your voice development journey.* Develop a practice of doing: voice responds to the 'little and often' principle of learning and adjustment. Develop a practice of listening: so much of voice development is the ability to listen to someone's voice and reflect 'ah, I know what's going on there.' Start with listening and tuning in to yourself – the development of your felt sense of voice (Mills & Pert, 2024; Mills & Stoneham, 2021; Morrison, 2022).

33 YOUR VOICE DEVELOPMENT IN ACTION

In the spirit of placing your voice process *first* and as the *bedrock* of vocal ethics, below is a guide to ingredients to include in regular practice. Make an 'unbreakable appointment with yourself' – that is, a commitment, a gift – of 30 minutes a couple of times a week to develop a rhythm of experiencing and discovery. Connect to an attitude of openness and play, allowing process itself to be the outcome. Inhabit the void, and invite becoming. Be curious and welcome the now and the new. You may wish to organise practice on your own and/or with fellow students, colleagues and friends in mutual support. In preparation, begin with quiet time to think about the following questions, designed to build a sense of your voice profile. Thereafter, move through the vocal workout, interweaving space to reflect on and journal your noticing. This is entirely the process, not necessarily the content, that we ask our clients to step into, as you will ask of your clients in time. Voice work is haptic and somatic, not intellectual and cerebral. Allow yourself to be warmly and mindfully with your perceptions and sensations without judgment. There are no 'right' answers towards a fixed map of the territory, but a myriad of possibilities in a landscape of potential. Allow destinations to shift and re-emerge as you are changed by the journey itself.

Know your voice:

- What do like and enjoy about your voice?
- What does your voice express with ease?
- What is challenging for your voice? Why?
- Who do you vocally admire, and who inspires you? How might you bring these qualities and features into your voice?
- What are the colours you can imagine in your voice?

- What are the elements you can imagine in your voice – earth, air, fire, water?
- How does your voice move through space?
- How and when are you vocally confident?
- How and when are you vocally vulnerable?
- How does anxiety affect your voice?
- How do you speak to loved ones, intimate partners, family members, friends, colleagues, authority figures, strangers, animals, yourself?
- How does your digital/telephone (audio only, non-visual cue) voice differ from your voice when people can see you?
- What are your social contexts and vocal code-switches?
- How do you project your voice and gain attention in noisy environments?
- What is your experience of performing and public speaking?
- Have you been misgendered with your voice? If so, how did you feel, and what did you do next?
- Have you consciously changed your voice to fit in?
- Have you ever felt like a vocal imposter?
- Who or what takes away your voice?
- How do you complain, protest, survive and thrive vocally?
- Do you enjoy accents and character voices? How do you play with changing your voice?
- How does your inner voice sound, your compassionate self?
- Do you sing in the shower? What do you sing?
- What is your relationship to silence?
- How are you seen and heard in the world?
- What name would give to the story of your voice so far?

Your regular practice check-list:

- **Grounding and aligning – balanced posture:**
    - Standing posture: aim for grounding, which is an even distribution of weight across both legs and feet, neither leaning back into your heels nor tipping forward into your toes.
    - Give yourself a spine which allows its s-shape, working to your own mobility and movement range.

- Sitting posture: rock your upper body forward and back gently from your hips to ensure you are neither collapsing your lower back nor pulling up with excess tension.
- **Stretching and releasing – free muscles:**
  - Freeing neck, shoulders, jaw, lips, base and body of tongue, rib cage.
  - Release of tension comes only through *release with breath*.
  - Release your knees so you are standing on the ground.
  - Release tightness in abdomen without letting your belly collapse and flop forward.
- **Awakening and extending – dynamic breath support:**
  - Semi-supine work on the floor.
  - Standing and sitting with alignment.
  - Let your breath 'drop' in to your abdomen.
  - Extend your breath capacity through /s/ out for count of 5–10–15–20.
- **Voicing and resonating – efficient voice production:**
  - Repeat your breath work replacing /s/ with /z/.
  - Ensure your larynx is not constricted.
  - Aim for voice flow and sending the sound out.
  - Develop your voice being forward on /u:/.
  - Travel through your whole range using 'ng', noticing your gear changes.
  - Hum an /m/ into your resonators – chest, throat, face, head.
  - Explore onsets of tone.
- **Playing and articulating – muscular diction:**
  - Consider using a bone prop to facilitate increased muscularity and vocal resonance (see Morrison, 2022).
  - Be playful and read a speech or poem (heightened language) that has significant meaning for you.

34 YOUR VOICE EXPANSION IN ACTION

Having profiled your voice, started to develop a regular practice, and tried out three important exercises, expand your voice further. Below are suggestions for vocal enquiries and experiments – your vocal project work. The aim is that this is ongoing work, not done once and put away – moving sound around, discovering new places and spaces, new light and shade, thickness and thinness, timbres and tones, codes and contexts.

- Explore amplifying, spreading, shifting, developing resonances without pushing or squeezing but through placing and sensing: chest, pharyngeal, facial, head.
- Make the sound of a duck, a trumpet, a child on a swing, a fire-engine, *Mars Attacks* aliens, a frog, a vibrating mobile phone – sense and feel into how you make these sounds. Make them bigger without pushing or straining.
- Use twang quality or facial placement/engagement for brightening.
- Use sternum placement/engagement for deepening/darkening.
- Explore using more expressive range in targeted speaking contexts.
- Explore prosody – emphasis and intonation – and the 'Laban of voice' (Mills & Stoneham, 2017).
- Develop a new code switch or distinct voice: observe imposter syndrome within you, and then give yourself total permission to be this new sound.
- Vary your launch pitch via thinking ('err'/'um') and agreeing sounds ('m-hm').
- Imitate cartoon and character voices – have fun.
- Explore making your sound less/more typically vocally gendered. What do you notice and how do you feel? Hold on to these sensations, insights and emotional reflections: they are gold dust.

35 AUTHOR DIALOGUE 'THE SPHERE AND THE CUBE'

Natasha: Yes, I really think that, without understanding these fundamental principles, it seems to me it is not possible to be an effective, sensitive, voice therapist, practitioner and coach to trans and non-binary people. Knowing what they mean, in a deep way, is part of developing an informed position that we write about in the first section.

Matthew: I have heard you speak often about vocal authenticity – finding what is vocally and uniquely you – can you say something about what that means to you in particular, Natasha?

Natasha: Yes, absolutely. So, it was an interesting journey in the sense that I realised, through the work we originally did together many years ago, that I didn't have to essentially change my voice – I had to actually *expand* it. If my voice were, let us say, the shape of a sphere, I didn't have to transform it into a cube. What I needed to do was to expand the sphere into a *bigger sphere* – one that could encompass more ways of expressing myself, and ultimately the ability to change the voice as well if required. And so, the process was an *expansion* of what was, not an erasure or replacement, but an *expansion*!

Matthew: You are saying that being authentic for you wasn't about cancelling or denying what is, but growing qualities or features within your sound, that you had taken through a kind of filtering process according to what was and is important to you, and then you expanded upon those qualities and features. And as you say, your voice ended up feeling, looking and perhaps sounding – different.

Natasha: Exactly – and my voice might have ended up sounding different, but it was a process of transformation, rather than a process of erasure and replacement. It wasn't a cancelling of something and the introduction of something else out of the blue, it was a transformation from one quality to another, through a gradual process that allowed my voice as a whole entity to change too.

Matthew: And a lot of this work over the years has been about *journeying* – going on a journey of discovery where you might start off heading for a destination that you have a strong idea about, but that your destination can and does change along the way because you are changed by the journey itself. Do you think that's right?

Natasha: Yes! A big part of it was *accepting* the fact that my voice sounded a certain kind of way, accepting that this was indeed the case; but then progressing towards changing it *enough* to sound in a way that felt comfortable, genuine and authentic to me and therefore to other people. So, it was the mix and balance of *acceptance and change*, at the same time, that were fundamental.

Matthew: I remember you saying clearly there was a certain moment where to do more change-orientated voice work would be adding to your dysphoria, because you knew that you had to be authentic with and about the features that you had in your voice. And that was a combination of both developing a voice and developing self-acceptance. These two trajectories are ones which seem opposed but are in fact deeply complementary and co-creative.

Natasha: Yes, exactly – not denying the part of me that will always be confined or limited by certain characteristics, maybe like geometry of the vocal cords or something.

Matthew: That's great, because you remind us of the truth that we none of us have one voice, but actually many voices. We have many relational codes we speak in many contexts – for example with our loved ones, and how our intimate voice is different to our voice or voices we use with our managers and colleagues at work.

Natasha: Yes, our assertive, professional voice may sound different to our sensual and sexual voices, or there may be some overlapping features.

Matthew: Yes, and how we speak to animals, how we talk to ourselves, how we sing, how we express love, desire, protest, how we speak on the phone – these are all part of us, aren't they? And this expansive, sphere of your voice holds all of those subtle and many spheres within it.

Natasha: We say to the reader, put your own voice journeying at the centre of your work to enable the journey of your trans and non-binary clients – and then you understand the vulnerabilities, the imposter syndrome, the challenges of practising, the potential horror of typical perceptions of gendered voice – and then you will not judge or other but allow your process to inform the process of your clients. This takes time – and you are at the beginning. Please give yourself time. Hurrying and rushing into pseudo expertise and professional status will do harm to your trans and non-binary clients.

Matthew: Thanks, Natasha. You're speaking deeply about what it is to be a vocal pedagogue – thank you.

36 MOTOR LEARNING PRINCIPLES

Motor learning principles inform effective pedagogy and foreground experiential processing. The more curious, motivated and autonomous we enable our clients to be in acquiring desired voice skills, the more creative, competent and enriched their sense of vocal self and journeying. Developing the client's awareness of physical sensations during voice work by engaging in *mindful enquiry* (Kabat-Zinn, 2016) about what they noticed, felt, heard, experienced *before* therapist feedback is absolutely key. Therapist demonstration of exercises is powerful and necessary in that it builds trust and collaboration, and we shine a light onto our processing, idiosyncrasy, potential vulnerability and modelling of transparency and self-compassion for imperfection in the moment. It is important to map exercise rationale to client goals, keeping analysis and instruction as brief, simple and concise as possible. When we give feedback, it is always honest about what we heard in relation to what was attempted. Praise is motivating ('Great, you had a go, you did it!') and momentary; constructive feedback extends perceptual learning and practice that is alive to sensing – 'What did you notice? What went well? What might you do more of next time?' We offer our therapist succinct feedback thereafter, free of judgment and overwhelming minutiae: 'I heard this. Try again, focussing on this ... ' Verdolini is a voice practitioner, researcher and experienced teacher who describes a model of 'Scan-Gel-Show-Tell' in building adroit perception (Titze & Verdolini, 2012). 'Scan' denotes mindful noticing (without changing) of body sensation and potential tension sights. 'Gel' denotes focused manipulation of a specific body part, muscle or vocal process. 'Show' refers to therapist demonstration. 'Tell' means giving instruction, and is best done as the final step, though this will depend somewhat on learning preference and whether the exercise or vocal behaviour is completely new.

37 PRACTICAL PEDAGOGY

Below are summaries of key pedagogical skills and processes that are useful to be *aware of*. Notice how voice coaches and teachers use them with you in your own voice development. With experience and time, we refine our own motivational style into that which is confident, supportive, clear and above all mindful (neither rushed nor delivered in automatic pilot).

- **Demonstrating** – therapist initiates (relational to client pitch and resonance profile).
- **Masking** (conjoining) – performing a vocal exercise in unison with the client.
- **Rhythmic scaffolding and turn-taking** – counting in ('after three … one, two, three'), gradating turn-taking towards client independence (e.g. 'my turn, turn together, my turn, turn together, my turn, your turn, turn together, your turn, your turn … ').
- **Contrastive practice** (e.g. contrasting launch pitch or resonance dial up/down) contrasting one voice parameter variable at a time enables *eureka* moments and lasting perceptual awareness (negative practice – contrasting to an undesired vocal behaviour – is best done only once due to the potential activation/increase of vocal dysphoria).

Related to The Drama Triangle, below are examples of coaching styles and the roles/positions that they map on to:

- **The defensive coach (Victim and Persecutor)**: watch the psychological and vocal transference and countertransference – if you are defensive and that leads you to over-explain and over-theorise, you will end up alienating the client.
- **The critical coach (Persecutor)**: watch your critical narrative in coaching and feedback and ensure frustration does

not leak out and demolish the client in their best attempt. If clients do not feel safe with you, you will not succeed in bringing anything out of them.
- **The coach who centres their process and talks too much (Victim and Rescuer)**: in teacher training this is referred to as 'TTT through the roof' – too much teacher talking time. Deft, emotionally processed, compassionate and discerning self-disclosure which illuminates some part of the client's journey and processing can be very powerful. But a coach that centres their own process to the detriment of the client's is inviting the energy flow towards themselves, the therapist, which is a subconscious request to be rescued. The client will politely accept in the first and second instances, but will soon disengage and ultimately feel angry and unseen – they will become the persecutor.
- **The compassionate and useful coach (Facilitator)**: this is meeting your client where they are, sensitively, in a trauma-informed and inclusive way that speaks to opening access needs; using a lot of masking and quick fire repetitions before much of the fear response has kicked in, diffuses anxiety, establishes trust and centres specificity.

38 HOW TO COACH AN EXERCISE

Following on from your understanding of motor learning and basic practical pedagogy above, here is the staged process to teaching/coaching your client into a new vocal exercise:

1. Very **briefly introduce an exercise** and say how it links to the client's goals and what it will enable. This allays fears and contains vocal dysphoria and lurking imposter syndrome.
2. Encourage the **client to be mindful** of their breathing and body in readiness to begin voice work – easy, relaxed and potent posture.
3. **Demonstrate** the exercise for the client.
4. Practise the pure exercise together with the client (**masking**) using a 'count in' ('and together, one, two, three ... ') – this is not bossy or chilly, but warm, strong, reassuringly

directive and supportive in the initial and early stages of practice.
5. **Practise the pure exercise** to encourage client independence, encouraging your client to develop how their larynx, throat, lips, face, chest, etc. and sense of flow *feel*. This is for perceptual awareness and confidence.
6. Add **cognitive-process consonance** by performing the exercise again with a description of what it is doing e.g. 'I am launching my voice at E3' while you are doing exactly that.
7. Perform the exercise as an **adaptation**, which begins to apply the skill to everyday speaking e.g. 'Err … I am looking out the window' (launching 'Err' at E3).
8. Increase skills of consciously **using adaptations in more specific and longer speaking situations**.

In a five-individual-session model, the first appointment is the scene-setting initial appointment. Thereafter the trajectory of four *therapy* sessions aims to embed the technical skills of using pitch, resonance, vocal fold weight/mass, intonation, leading the client to be able to practise independently, to self-monitor, to self-correct, to self-select accurate pitch launching according to their goals and practice, to use story intonation (e.g. 'three things I did this morning'; 'I went to the supermarket and bought … '), and to use expressive intonation and bounces (Mills & Stoneham, 2021). After individual sessions, your client can progress to voice groups which aim to practise skills in more complex speaking situations (phone work, presentations and story-telling, voice projection, presence, assertiveness, embodiment) and to centre community support, wisdom and feedback.

39 AUTHOR DIALOGUE 'IMPOSTER SYNDROME TO VOCAL BELONGING'

Matthew: I think understanding *vocal othering* is so key for me. Nobody wants to feel like they are putting on a voice because that feels 'other', 'imposter', 'fake.' The very process of voice exploration makes people aware – literally self-conscious – and that can activate and trigger more vocal gender dysphoria.

Natasha: Yes, because it makes people more aware, yes. Awareness has to become absorbed.

Matthew: And we steer our clients through this, so that they can integrate, absorb – yes, I like that, Natasha – and celebrate new vocal qualities. We have to be self-conscious of developing new skills in order to expand them and move in and out of unconscious processing and competence.

Natasha: The 'conscious-competence' model is such a helpful construction for all of us!

Matthew: It is important to hold all the vocal possibilities of being human in us, not a slim version of gendered voice solely related to cisnormative performance, and enable the client to give themselves permission to have their own voice-scape, their own shifts, code-switches and plural vocal identities, their own perceptions of gendered voice, their own strategies to meet normative and typically perceived vocal expectations in order to feel safe or congruent.

Natasha: Helping clients find voicing that is intrinsic and not 'fancy dress.' It takes practice, guidance and belief in ourselves, belief in our ability to play and become. I like the analogy of a new hairstyle – on the first day we had the new style, we can feel self-conscious and maybe a few people notice the change, but after a while, nobody notices the change, and people acclimatise to our new state, and that becomes the default – in us and for people around us.

Matthew: We are helping to bring voicing and voices *home* – they are not out there, but in here, and they belong, they are not other and weird, we claim them, and we know them, and they are ours.

Natasha: So, Matthew, we have vocal othering and the impact of imposter syndrome, softening and becoming vocal integration, celebration and belonging. It is doable!

40 THE INITIAL APPOINTMENT

The initial therapist–client meeting in trans voicing therapy is an information giving-and-gathering *appointment*, not an assessment. The main purpose is to establish the therapeutic contract and way of working, to hear the client's voice likes and challenges; vocal comfort rating; physical and psychological well-being and levels of social support; voice experimentation and exploration to date; voice goals and access needs, to give information about voice therapy as a process and how to practice; and to make an agreed plan for the next appointment. We want to try to arrive at the question 'how can I help you?' as early as possible in the session.

Here is a summary of items to aim to include in your initial appointment:

- Introductions – name and pronouns – therapist-initiated.
- Therapeutic contract and way of working – confidentiality, safeguarding, expertise, number of sessions, process of voice change, no expectations or assumptions.
- Checking client access needs and learning preferences.
- Your transparent positionality: authentic and unique voicing, relation to normativity.
- Brief information gathering of hydration, smoking, vaping, hay fever, asthma, reflux, hormones (if pertinent – such as problems starting, GP support, commencement of t, length of time on t).
- Checking client emotional well-being and social support.
- Understanding client goals – **'how can I help you?'**
- Client 'communication map' (voice codes and contexts), vocal comfort rating, likes, concerns.
- Summarising and confirming goals, then *brief* vocal explanation of voice/pitch/resonance/vocal fold weight.
- Vocal try-outs: matching pitch, resting pitch, raising launching pitch (High-Bright-Thin), establishing lower pitch range (Low-Chest-Thick), contrasting resonance, contrasting vocal fold weight (depends on client).
- Feedback: 'what went well and what are you pleased to notice?'

- Clarifying practice: apps to download and use, exercises, practice specifics (of what, how, how often, when, where), noticing and journalling progress.
- Confirming therapy plan going forward and booking in next appointment.

Depending on your client, some of the above items will take more time (you may need to come back to some in a second session), and some will need to be touched upon only briefly. Know why you are asking *everything* you ask of your client, and be transparent about your rationale for doing so. It is a consultative dialogue, not a shopping list or automated script – which would feel tedious and lifeless for both you and your client.

41 AUTHOR DIALOGUE 'MEETING WITH THE CLIENT'

To breathe further life into key point 40 above, we enacted a role play of the first part of an initial voice therapy appointment, transcribed below, as an example and guide, only. Keep constantly in mind that you aim to meet the client where they are in every aspect of your interaction.

Matthew: Hello, I'm Matthew, the pronouns that I use are he/him, and sometimes they/them. Welcome to this speech and language therapy appointment about your voice. First of all, can I check, what you would like me to call you?

Natasha: Oh, hi, Matthew, thanks, nice to meet you. Please call me Natasha.

Matthew: Thanks so much, Natasha, and can I ask what pronouns you use?

Natasha: My pronouns are she and her.

Matthew: Thanks for letting me know. Welcome to this this initial appointment. You've spoken to one of my colleagues about your voice and been referred to me.

So, the purpose of our appointment today is an opportunity for me to hear from you the things you might be thinking about with your voice, what's important to you about your voice, things you enjoy about your voice, things you might be worrying about with your voice, things you may want to explore with your voice. It's an opportunity for me to explain what voice work is, what we do, how we do it, how many sessions I can give you, what the process is, so that by the end of today's session, we'll have a plan together. We may do some voice work today if that fits with you, so you have some practical work to take away with you from today. Does that sound ok?

Natasha: Yes, that sounds really fine.

Matthew: And if there's anything that I say or ask that you're not sure about, please just stop me and say 'Matthew, I don't know why you're asking that.' Because this session is for you and I am in service of you.

Natasha: That makes me feel less nervous – thanks.

Matthew: I also want to say right up front, and we say this to all of our patients who see us in speech and language therapy, that there is absolutely no expectation on my part or my colleagues' part that you have to change or explore your voice. We start with the premise, and truth, that everyone has a totally authentic and individual voice (even voices), that there are as many feminine voices as there are women, as many masculine voices as there are men, and as many non-binary voices as there are non-binary people. Everyone's voice and voicing is completely unique! There are no stereotypes here, and we're here to help you to find your authentic voicing. And maybe you have found this already. Does that make sense?

Natasha: Yes, that really helps to know that.

Matthew: Before we get started with the details about your voice, let me also confirm that this is a confidential space and what we talk about stays with us in this room. I am part of the gender team and that means that if there is something you tell me that makes me think you need more support than I can give you, either from your GP or the gender team, then we can talk about that and I can take it to the team. We are here to support you and how you are doing with exploration. Would you say transition?

Natasha: Yes, transition is a word that I use. Ok, thank you, I understand that.

Matthew: Can I also ask if you have particular access needs and learning preferences, and how you want me to present any information?

Natasha: Yes, I like to understand concepts and have information in visual form then follow instruction or a demonstration.

Matthew: Thanks for letting me know. Whatever exercises we do, I'll explain what they do for your voice, demonstrate them and show you how to do them, then we'll do them together, so you can feel how they are for you, and practise them at home on your own. You are an expert in your voice and voicing – you may not know that yet – but you are – and you have your experience of the sound. I am expert in my voice and voicing, and I am still learning, and I have an expertise in *voice work* – and between us, our shared expertise comes together so that you can become conscious and competent with your voice work from your internal experience and from my feedback as an external ear. Does that make sense?

Natasha: Yes, I think that's clear. It's helping me feel less nervous all the time.

Matthew: So, let's start. A few brief questions first of all – things I ask about because they can affect your voice – do you or have you ever smoked or vaped?

Natasha: I used to smoke a lot when I was younger, but I haven't smoked in almost 11 years. I don't vape.

Matthew: Thanks. Do you ever suffer from heartburn or acid reflux as we call it?

Natasha: I have suffered from it at times if I eat just before bed. Sometimes it happens, but not on a daily basis. And I haven't had it for a long while now.

Matthew: Yes, important to allow at least a couple of hours after eating and going to bed, so we're not actively digesting food when we lie down. Any hay fever or asthma?

Natasha: No, no, I don't have them. And I'm not allergic to pollen or anything like that.

Matthew: Thanks for letting me know. And how's your daily hydration – when you go to the loo, is your pee pale in colour?

Natasha: You ask that because being hydrated helps my voice?

Matthew: Yes, it's like putting oil in a car engine – keeps things running smoothly. No need to be gulping water – but more about keeping your systemic, body hydration topped up and optimum throughout the day.

Natasha: I see yes, I think it's fine – I drink about a litre and a half of water throughout the day. I don't drink coffee anymore.

Matthew: You're really on top of that. And I can hear your voice is really well produced. Lastly, I know you are well established on your hormones – I just want to check – do you have a supportive GP and are you on top of getting your bloods done regularly?

Natasha: Yes, I have been on feminising hormones for several years – oestrogens, and my GP is adequate.

Matthew: Thanks for answering these questions, Natasha. So – now – *how can I help you?*

Natasha: Oh, thank you so much. Okay, so I wanted to come and see you as a specialist, because I'm a transgender woman, and I'm in the process of transitioning. And I have made great progress in the way that I present myself visually, but not so much progress in the way that I sound. And I feel like I sound a little bit more masculine than I would like to, when I hear my voice on a recording. I don't necessarily like my voice – the sound of my voice – at the moment. I don't think it fits with my presentation. I've tried to use a couple of apps but I found them difficult to work with, and many have a very prescriptive and narrow sense of what gendered voice is, and that seems very cis informed, and that's not helpful to me. So, I thought that I needed more specialist help, that I needed face to face, specialist help. And that's why I'm here.

Matthew: Thank you so much for this, that's really helpful for me to understand where you're coming from. Yes, apps can be useful, the ones that give you a practice note, or give you information about your starting pitch, or your pitch range, or the expressive up and down of your voice, which we call intonation. But mostly voice work is best done in the room or remotely by Zoom if the therapist is experienced – as an *interactive* process. It's about muscle training and motor learning. It's about exploration and a journey together. Can I ask – what do you like about your voice? What do you most enjoy about the way you communicate?

Natasha: I hadn't thought you would ask that, but good that you have. Well, I generally like my voice as a tool. I like the way I sound to others, and their response to how I speak. But not necessarily the fabric of my voice. I like the fact that I can be assertive, I can sound assertive. I work as a therapist currently and I have worked in advertising. I attended frequent board meetings. I can be quite an assertive person. I can project my voice well; I can sound quite authoritative at times if I wanted to. But what I don't like is how the fabric of the voice is a little bit too masculine, in my ears anyway. So, I like the effect of my voice and the impact of it as a communication tool. Which is great. I love it. Because it sounds like me, it is me. But I'm not sure how it sounds, fully.

Matthew: So, you generally like how you sound to others, you like that you can project your voice and be assertive, but you don't like how the *fabric* of your voice sounds a little too masculine to you. Is that right?

Natasha: Yes, that's it.

Matthew: Can you tell me more about the fabric of your voice, and what words would you use to describe how you'd like your voice to feel and sound to you?

Natasha: Absolutely. Yes, the fabric. I think that I don't want to fully change my voice per-se, I want to improve my ability to sound closer to how I feel about myself. So, if for example one day I feel very feminine, I can wear a dress – a sun dress if it's hot, and heels or whatever, and go out. And I feel quite feminine in my body and my presentation. I want to be able to do the same with my voice. If I feel like I want to sound feminine in a particular situation, or more feminine than I do at the moment, I want to be able to expand my voice to accommodate that option.

Matthew: What you are touching on, I think, is that we all have many voices and our voice changes depending who we are speaking to, the context, the situation – it's authentic to have many voices, however subtle the differences are, and we change up and down these subtle gears – our vocal code-switches. We can have a *home* place in our voice and we shift from there by bringing out certain features like pitch or tone/timbre; some people have quite distinct separate vocal identities which represent different aspects of themselves. This is all well. So, we're not eradicating or cancelling our voice but foregrounding certain features more, *filtering* them, so there's no judgment of your voice as it is now, and we embrace our voice today and, as best we can, celebrate it and mould it into change with as much gentle care and compassion as we can muster.

Natasha: I love that, yes.

Matthew: Let's begin some voice work. Let's begin by establishing what your resting pitch is – that easy mid-low place in your voice, and if you feel that raising it to a comfortable degree so it starts a little higher is something that feels right, then knowing the resting pitch will be useful to see where we want to lift it. OK?

Natasha: Yes

Matthew: So, I'd like you to count one to ten quite slowly, about this sort of pace (demonstrated one number per second), using your voice absolutely as you have been talking to me now, not trying to change anything. I will listen (if on Zoom – put myself on mute) and use my perfect piano keyboard app to match your pitch without disturbing you, and then we'll see together if you agree and that feels about right.

Natasha: OK here goes, one, two, three, four, five, six, seven, eight, nine, ten.

Matthew: OK so I heard you starting your 'one' around F3, then you stepped down, as we tend to, towards your finishing note on 'ten' ending around B2. We use these musical names as short hand for the amount of vibrations per second – so F3 is 175Hz (your vocal folds coming together 175 times per second to make that particular pitch), and B2 is 123.5Hz. Amazing because you started the sound, you launched your speaking from F3, and this is in what we would call a 'typically perceived feminine pitch according to a general public used to a cisnormative sound.' That sounds like a mouthful, but I am being careful about my words.

Natasha: I understand exactly what you mean and thanks for being sensitive. It's the perception of the public – a normative based sound expectation, within a kind of a range.

Matthew: Yes, and given that you want to increase your sense of achieving a more feminine sound in certain social contexts, let's use the wisdom of what your voice is already doing by helping it achieve a more consistent launch around F3. From there, we can bring in and play with what we call 'brightening resonance' and 'thinning' the voice. We can touch on what these words mean, before starting to do some launching pitch exercises at F3 …

Natasha: Yes, thanks, that's good …

42 HIGH-BRIGHT-THIN THERAPY

Figure 8.1 is a schema which describes therapy focused towards vocal skills (single and combined) – raising launching pitch to a comfortable and achievable degree, brightening and forward-placing resonance, and thinning vocal fold weight/mass. This is what we used to describe as voice feminisation and now refer to as 'High-Bright-Thin.' This is because terminology which centres the therapy and skill focus rather than gender identity

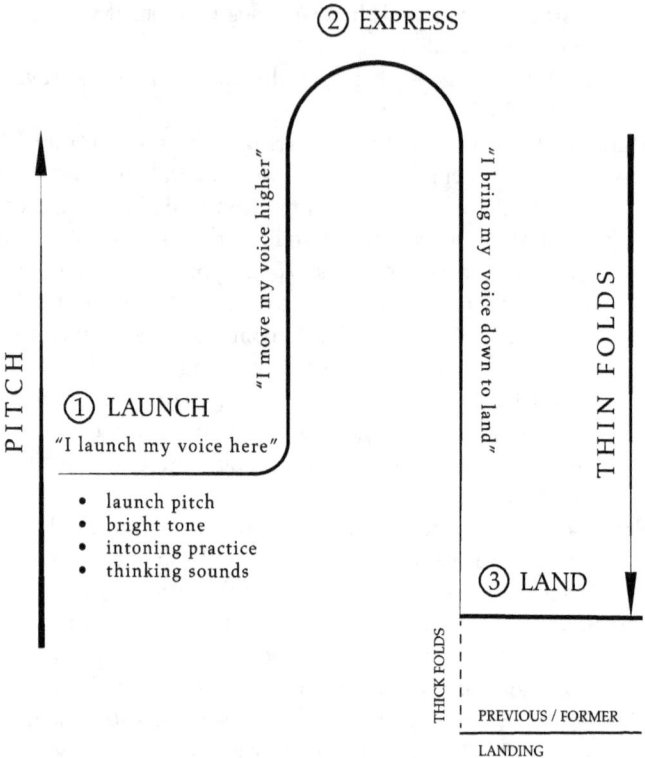

Figure 8.1 Launch-Express-Land for High-Bright-Thin Voice Work

is more open and inclusive to clients exploring a range and mix of characteristics. Moreover, therapy-specific nomenclature off-sets and makes conscious potential cisnormative bias and fixed ideas of what 'feminine' voice is, whilst acknowledging a common set of skills clients tell us are important to them (Mills & Pert, 2024). Detailed descriptions of vocal exercises are not part of this text; however, we summarise the essentials below for your orientation.

As you are learning from the introduction to pedagogy above, in the **first step** of vocal work, it is vital not to block the client's access to their perceptual training and initial tuning into sensation by over analysis. Absolutely at the outset we must allay fears of imposter syndrome and sensitively navigate gender vocal dysphoria by the briefest introduction to exercises and how their rationales link to client goals. Then, we are straight into the pure exercises, experiencing them, tuning into and sensing them. What we then find to be powerful for clients as a **second step** is to perform the exercise again, both practising *and* describing the skill simultaneously – what they are doing while they are doing it. This is **cognitive-process consonance**. It helps to steer practice, make voice work more concrete, and speed development. Build perceptual relationship to new experience first, then you can combine sensing and descriptive processing, helpfully. Hence: 'I launch my voice here' refers to the intoning work that has been focused to D3, E3, F3, G3. 'I move my voice higher' refers to allowing vocal intonation to move according to personal communicative intention – i.e. it moves from intoning into intonational contour. It also focuses the client to aim for the bright resonance right at the onset of speaking. 'I bring my voice down to land' refers to the work of thinning vocal fold posture 'all the way to the bottom of my voice' so that clients land with definite confidence without travelling to a lower pitch range in thick vocal fold posture.

Let us be clear about what we mean by **vocal exercises** and **adaptations**. Vocal exercises are those behaviours we practise in pure form – humming at pitch, intoning at pitch, resonance contrast, intoning into speaking, thickening and thinning vocal fold posture. Adaptations are brief speaking activities which deliberately translate an exercise into an everyday conversational unit or activity. For example, intoning at E3 and launching E3 becomes the adaptation of a thinking sound 'err/um' at E3 which launches a sentence. So, **mmm12345 at E3** becomes 'Err [intoned at E3] ... my favourite colour is green.' Another adaptation is the **lengthened 'I' or 'I'm.'** So, mmm12345 at E3 becomes '**I'm ... [lengthened and intoned at E3]** ... looking out the window.'

What the Launch-Express-Land model also offers is a sense of vocal spatial awareness. It offers a kind of *vocal geography* which consciously refers to pitch in its construct of 'up and down' related spatially to higher and lower than the horizon line or height of the client. It is important to note, also, that 'high' in and of itself is meaningless. When we learn music, and there is a dynamic marking of 'p' (*piano*, meaning soft/quiet in Italian), we ask ourselves 'quieter than what?' In the same way, **'high' means higher than the resting pitch.** That is why we start with the counting to discover the resting pitch, which turns out to be not too far away from the launching pitch to be established – and needs to be a process which starts close to the resting pitch, likely around C3 and D3, then steps up to E3 and F3. F3# and G3 might be desirable and attainable by the client – in which case, fantastic. It may be, for example, important to be able to launch higher on the phone. But watch out for thoughts that 'the higher the better.' If we push the launch pitch as high as possible, we end up with a high, flat voice, which sounds unbalanced and has within it a fear of coming down and landing. Ultimately, the launch and land place become the most important aspects of this work. We start with pitch work because raising pitch is the single most difficult thing to habituate in a new voicing pattern. There is a current trend in anecdotal comment and generalisation by inexperienced voice therapists or non-voice colleagues that 'it's not all about pitch.' Well, that is partially correct, but discounting the importance of pitch work is bunkum. Competent gender-affirming voice therapy is about pitch work that is *absolutely specific* and without that, no matter how much skill the client has to brighten resonance and thin vocal fold posture, the overall effect may be disappointing to them, especially if the aim is to sound more 'typically perceived as vocally feminine by the general public.' The lack of specificity of pitch work is an indication of the therapist's is inexperience – this is why we start with relational pitch work in therapist training and vocal processing.

Crucially, *Launch-Express-Land* can facilitate many learning preferences – especially visual and kinaesthetic approaches. These are both enormously helpful to integrate into your demonstration and scaffolding of an exercise, consonance and adaptation – so long as you are not generalising in shape and that every part of your hand gesture, movement and flow manifests the intonational contour, and describes the interrelationship between the top of speaking voice, the bottom of speaking voice and where the launch place is, and the quality of *flow* of voicing from lips to listener/spot on the wall/target of sound. If we generalise in our demonstration, we lead the client to exercise inaccuracy, sensory confusion and cognitive-process dissonance, which, unacknowledged, leads to the breakdown in the therapeutic and coaching relationship. The greatest damage that we can do as a vocal coach is to give inaccurate or false feedback and let ourselves vocally rescue because we are overwhelmed with our client's anxiety or frustration. Stay present, mindful and compassionate. There is always the chance to have another go. If your forte is not with kinaesthetic gestural cuing (it has to be practised in pedagogical training), simply own that and foreground visual cues and representation – perhaps based on the schema visual as well as the client's individual visual/image. Clients have spoken of launching as like 'posting a letter' and 'choosing which diving board to jump off'; expressing as if 'going up and over a hill' and 'skipping or jumping along'; and landing as though 'putting the breaks on gently as I drive down a hill and come to a stop at the bottom' and 'parachuting down to land and landing easily on my feet.' Discover – in time – your clients' rich description, images, metaphors and similes – whatever makes personal sense for each.

- **Launch**
  - **Pure exercise**: humming a pitch, intoning a sequence, initiating bright tone (Mills & Pert, 2024) ('smile' tone – Mills & Stoneham, 2017).
  - **Cognitive-process consonance**: 'I launch my voice here' (intoned).
  - **Adaptation**: agreeing sound 'm-hm', 'u-huh' (where the 'm' and the 'u' are at launch pitch); 'Err, Umm, So, Well, So-erm, Well-erm, And-erm' thinking sounds at launch pitch; lengthened 'I' and 'I'm' into a sentence of what you are doing, seeing right now.

- **Express**
  - **Pure exercise**: intoning into speaking, following through with bright tone; contrast of resonance (home, dial up/down – Mills & Pert, 2024).
  - **Cognitive-process consonance**: 'I move my voice higher.'
  - **Adaptation**: continuation of a phrase or sentence launched by a thinking sound, an agreeing sound 'm-hm', 'u-huh' and 'yes'; phrases which have launch and bounce.
- **Land**
  - **Pure exercise**: 'ah' slide thin folds from top of speaking voice to bottom of new landing place which sounds intentionally and communicatively finished – the full stop; contrast of thin and thick vocal fold posture.
  - **Cognitive-process consonance**: 'I bring my voice down to land'; 'I am speaking in my thin voice all the way down to the bottom of my voice.'
  - **Adaptation**: continuation of a phrase or sentence launched and expressed, focussing on the satisfaction of completion: 'I'm ... looking out of the window'; 'Err ... my favourite season is summer'; 'Well, we had a brilliant time at the weekend'; 'I ... want to speak to the manager'; 'I'm ... getting ready to go out'; etc.

43 LOW-CHEST-THICK THERAPY

Figure 8.2 is the schema which describes the therapy focus of embodiment – developing resonance which is connected easily into the chest, sternum base of skull and pharynx, and layers up easily into face and head resonances. This focus of skills is entered into by clients wanting to deepen voice – some taking testosterone, and others not. Principally, the way forward is more what we call traditional performance-based voice work – where we are laying the foundations of aligned body, dynamic breath support, easy voice production, larynx deconstructed for tone onset, vocal fold closure efficient and flexible across full surface area to thinner contact, and articulation which is strong and free. Many people who start on t find that the

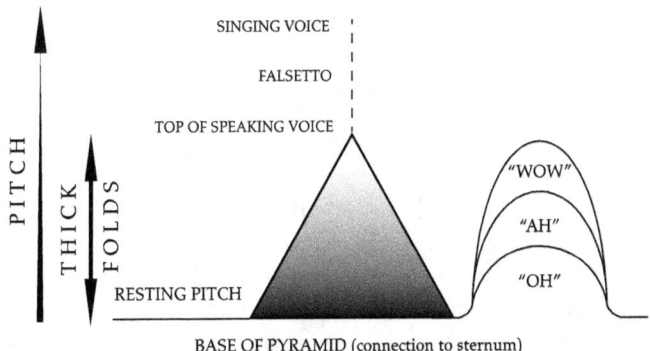

Figure 8.2 Low-Chest-Thick (Embodiment) Voice Work

lack of change in the vocal tract together with the thickening of the vocal folds is difficult to manage, especially when there is an identity memory of a voice with higher-brighter-thinner characteristics. There is some similarity in physical holding pattern, though **not** psychological processing, with adolescent puberphonia with cis young men. It is worth noting that there is a much greater commonality and shared experience of vocal growth with t between cis and trans people than has been noted. This is not in any way to discount the gender dysphoria of trans people taking t, this is to humanise the shared challenges that voices experiencing growth with testosterone undergo.

We cannot develop chest resonance by pushing or shoving the voice down. Wise and profound voice teacher, Cicely Berry, used to describe resonance as the quality which draws the listener in (Berry, 1994). We have to gather resonance, sense and grow the vibrations and let them amplify in our resonant spaces and travel through our bones according to the process of osteophony – literally allowing the bones to sound, to sing (Morrison, 2022). Think of the movement of water beginning as a trickle through a new landscape. Water finds a path that, once initiated, is followed and habituated and amplified with the increase of volume and pressure. Resonance is remarkably similar. In voicing therapy if we touch and place resonance, the regular sensing and awareness of it in different bones and spaces will lead to its development, amplification and growth. This is what we mean by sternum hook up – placing the embodiment of our resonance in the sternum and manubrium, like the base of a pyramid (see schema). This means that we can develop vocal fold closure and thick vocal fold posture in our lowest pitches, and maintain that all the way up to the top of our speaking voice without cracking or 'getting stuck' or 'squeaking.' However, we do not push thick folds beyond the passaggio, gear change or trap door which takes us into falsetto. Navigation of speaking voice into the singing voice and vice versa is beyond the scope of this text and orientation for the beginner. Speech and language therapists who are trained singers or have a solid singing technique can advise clients on this aspect of the work – in conjunction with the client's singing gender-sensitive teacher. Kaidyn Hinds, award winning professional singer, has been a great pioneer of this collaborative work (Mills & Pert, 2024). Developing thick vocal folds has brought images of bowling your voice (Boston, 2018).

- **Pure exercise**: 'ah slide' to establish lowest pitch (evidence of growth on t); 'ah' slide contrast thick and thin vocal posture; three circles siren to explore the whole range (Mills & Pert, 2024); chest sensing/tapping; skull sensing; jaw shake; tongue base stretch; clock-face drop; rib stretches.
- **Cognitive-process consonance**: 'I'm speaking in my thick voice all the up and down.'
- **Adaptations**: 'Oh', 'Ah', 'Wow', keeping connected to sternum. Repeating to sentence level: 'oh, that's great'; 'ah, I understand now'; 'wow, you look amazing in that!' 'wow, that's incredible!' 'Err/Um' in thick folds at low launching pitch; 'm-hm' and 'u-huh' agreeing sounds in low launching pitch with thick folds.

44 NON-BINARY VOICING

Non-binary voicing is as varied as there are non-binary people. Some non-binary people may want to occupy a pitch range and resonance profile that feels androgynous to them. Many clients have what we call mixed goals for voice – that is, creating and sustaining a bespoke vocal profile. What is common is the sense that clients often want to move away from a sound related to a pre-transition gender history. Therapists need to be sensitive about eliciting this; it probably straightforward to know if the vocal folds were exposed to testosterone in adolescent puberty or not, and go from there. Many non-binary people who did not have vocal fold growth significantly in adolescent puberty do not wish to take testosterone, and therefore pitch lowering must be semi-tonal only and minimally lower than the resting pitch, elicited by counting.

We commence goals which centre alleviation of vocal gender dysphoria and then move on to what brings the client vocal euphoria. This means that we enable the client to develop features so that people cannot gender their voice typically. We work on each parameter discretely – pitch, resonance, vocal fold weight – and you keep one stable and then play around with contrasting the others and find something that feels right for the client. This might become the client's 'all the time voice' or your home place voice, and then they observe specific parameters for certain code switches to navigate specific social/vocal situations – and then they become a pattern or bespoke combination through the day.

Clients have described non-binary voice work as finding authentic voicing, exploring multidimensional space of voices, varying voice over the course of a conversation or even phrase, controlling the impulse to 'correct' up or down, feeling you are out of your comfort zone or just at the zone of proximal development, and gradually moving back or side to side. In fact, such rich description is not simply about non-binary voices, but about the diversity of voices in general. Contrast is everything. Giving permission for code switching and voicing pluralities is incredibly important.

45 THE A + B = C OF PRACTICE

If you practised pure exercises for five minutes a day, would you notice voice change? The answer is yes, but progress would be slow. There needs to be a transparent description of the process of praxis. Here is the A + B = C process:

1. Start with practising the pure exercise(s) [**A**].
2. Straight afterwards, practise the adaptations of the pure exercise(s) [**B**].
3. Throughout the day, consciously bring in adaptions into everyday speech [**C**].

This is a conscious competence process. Eventually, the adaptations will become automatic, and the client will be able to rehearse silently, to hear voice in their head as their new default voice. There is a maxim in voice work which approximates as follows: the regular practice you do today will be felt and benefited by you in four months in terms of being integrated into conscious and sometimes unconscious competent voice use.

Encourage your client to practise **quick win warm-ups** into adaptations in the morning, then brought into speech consciously throughout the day:

1. Morning: practise the exercises + practise the adaptations.
2. In the day: find moments consciously to bring in the adaptations into everyday talking.
3. In the day: find time consciously to use the scripts in specific contexts.
4. In the day: disguise practice of adaptations by pretending to be speaking to someone on the phone.
5. At the end of the day: journal what went well; review your exercises and adaptations. Enjoy the power and self-gift of the process.

46 POPULATION CONSIDERATIONS

Notwithstanding that every client is unique, and you will need to adapt to their access needs, here are a number of potential population profiles to keep in mind.

- **Ageing larynx** – when a client has presbyphonia and/or significant lack of flexibility (perhaps related to scarring from phonosurgery or damage caused by nodules, Reinke's oedema, etc.), neither push down to a strained lower pitch, nor push up to an unsustainable and uncomfortable launching pitch range (C3# or D3 is more likely to be comfortable);

- **Young people** – voices still growing need careful handling; start with the effects of stress on voice, develop confidence in social communication, progress to specific gender voicing exercises and code-switches; honour the young person's expertise (Mills & Stoneham, 2021).
- **Stress and social anxiety** – mindfulness, deconstriction, small victories.
- **Singers and performers** – steam inhalation, vocal flow and navigation of passaggios, confidence in speaking voice range, extending speaking into singing, re-finding range with different voice qualities and resonances; work in liaison with a gender-affirming and experienced singing teacher.
- **People not taking t** – resonance development and semitone only shift downwards in pitch.
- **Phono surgical clients** – ensure voice therapy has maximised potential; ensure deconstriction is a known state; honour body autonomy of client while checking that client does not expect vocal panacea with surgery; work sensitively to uncover the extent of internalised transphobia with voice; ENT surgical providers must organise pre- and post-SLT/voice measurements and aftercare. If you work in the NHS, voice surgery is not commissioned, and so the whole package of phonosurgery intervention and management needs to be carried out by the private ENT clinical team.

47 AUTHOR DIALOGUE 'OUTCOMES THAT MATTER'

Matthew: Accountable services and practitioners must demonstrate that we are providing high quality and effective care. Therapy outcome measures are important in showing a basic pre-post therapy shift in the client's progress.

This will be primarily in their sense of their voice – technical skill, vocal comfort, vocal euphoric moments, confidence in using voice in easy and challenging situations, resilience and vocal victories.

Natasha: Yes, and trans voicing – needs to have client outcomes at the centre, which are definitely not brought in from pathology models. I have heard of something called the voice handicap index. I don't think I want to be answering questions on that!

Matthew: Professionally, speech and language therapy outcome measures and questionnaires have tended to be constructed around deficit and impairment.

Natasha: But we have done work, and you have done work in voice groups co-produced with your clients about their *journey of voice*, its development – well-being scores, new stories about what we have learned, new skills, the challenges overcome, the support. I remember it well.

Matthew: Yes, you helped develop questions from pilot groups in our service in London. So, we use a simple client self-rated voice comfort scaling, in-house questionnaires developed from the community about voice groups, and the Journey of Voice Development, based on Michael White's Narrative Therapy work on the stages of journeying to new vocal 'places.'

Natasha: We did a lot of work literally putting that on the map.

Matthew: Thank you, Natasha. And have we missed anything? What constitutes a good voice outcome for you? What more could therapists be doing and capturing?

Natasha: Well, capturing progress in developments in technique, application and support. They are vital. Good outcomes for me are also ones that are both open-ended and boundaried in some senses. So, they don't and must not look in a particular rigid way – it's not a conveyor belt – but they also have something tangible to capture. Therefore, a good outcome will look different for every client that comes through your door, and they are measured against the client's very personal and particular goals they came in with or have reviewed along the way, and have arrived at now. That seems obvious to say.

Matthew: But absolutely worth saying – thanks.

Natasha: And I suppose there are those definite parameters like the pitch that someone is starting with and moving to – the launching pitch as we say – those are easily measureable and helpful quantitative data, so long as it describes the personal journey of the client and what we feel success in. A pitch launch change of 10Hz may be amazing for client A, and change of 20Hz for client B may be disappointing, so we are all different. Capture our stories in how we use our voices. And let our stories be our own about our progress, not somehow hijacked in professional circles to advertise the reputation of the therapist. We need you to ask us for dynamic consent in our absence. But, yes, our successes, confidence – a mixture of qualitative and quantitative measures. And questionnaires, if we must have them, to be designed by the people with lived experience from the outset of the design process.

Matthew: That's really clear, Natasha. We learn so much from you, always.

Natasha: For me – we discussed this earlier – that a good outcome was for me to *expand* my voice and to have skills in particular settings that I could use in other times when I felt comfortable to display more of me, to show more of me, when I'd be using a different style of voice, such as on the phone. I would use specific skills to not be misgendered, to be understood, to get my point across at a meeting at work – to project my voice; to use my voice in intimate contexts authentically, to be assertive and expressive.

Matthew: Celebrating the flexibilities of your voice, and accepting where it is today and its potential in the future.

Natasha: Yes, outcomes that matter and are meaningful have to link to acceptance overall – acceptance of what the voice is like and sounds like in relationship to the whole person, to the identity of the person. So, ultimately, the outcome with most meaning is to feel *congruent* in my voice.

Matthew: Many clients talk about consistency, and I ask them – consistency of what? Being more specific in the goal and therefore in the outcome.

Natasha: Yes, and of course consistency is important in that we want to rely on our skills and vocal competence. For example, it plays a role when we are asked our name or a 'regular' type question about ourselves, we want to respond easily in a way without thinking about it – automatically, so that we are able to respond with an unconscious competency in a way that is consistent and you are not afraid of what will come out. It has happened to me a lot in recent years when I have been very comfortable in using my voice and the desired effect is there – there's a consistent vocal identity that I am using. That takes some time, but I think everyone wants to get to a place where they just want to speak with a voice they are happy with and can rely on. And being specific about consistency certainly helps, for sure.

Chapter 9

SUMMARY – THE TRANS-AFFIRMATIVE SLT

> **OVERVIEW**
> - This chapter aims to summarise the core discussion of professional status quo, and conclude with affirmations and learning statements to guide the reader's onward journey and progress through trans cultural humility, lifelong vocal apprenticeship, coaching and pedagogical practice, therapeutic skill and psychological mindedness, authentic positionality.
> - It contains Key Points 48–50.

48 PROFESSION IN CRISIS?

There is a labour shortage in the UK's National Health Service (NHS Scotland, NHS England, NHS Wales, and Health and Social Care of Northern Ireland), and currently 20% of speech and language therapy posts are not filled. The removal of NHS bursaries for degree courses and registration training for speech and language therapists signals a less diverse and less buoyant student intake. We need to support the profession and galvanise NHS trusts to increase creation of internships and technical assistant and speech and language therapy assistant posts which encourage and enable applicants from marginalised communities, especially people of colour and gender diverse people, to gain the necessary experience to apply for registration degrees into the profession. It is unfortunate that restrictions in free movement of people post-Brexit and the UK's decision not to take part in the Erasmus+ programme as a Programme Country have radically reduced the number of exchange projects and educational opportunities to welcome students from within the European Member states.

Simply, there are not enough gender specialist, trans-affirmative clinicians in the field to meet the current demand. There is a growing, enthusiastic new generation of SLTs coming into the field, but without trained voices, green in clinical voice disorders and naive in non-pathology voice work and pedagogy. The catastrophic wait times of between 23 and 87 months for first appointments at gender services (www.genderkit.org.uk) force many trans people to seek expensive consultations in private healthcare, for which there is little health insurance and from which a great many trans and non-binary people are excluded due to the financial barriers of living in significant poverty. It is a step in the right direction that NHS England has commissioned more 'pilot' clinics to become part of the constellation of permanent gender services. However, there is a dearth of suitably vocally trained and skilled SLTs currently, and it takes several years to develop and hone vocal practice. We know that it is unethical to work beyond our scope of practice and competence. Our professional and regulatory bodies warn that it is inadvisable, even potentially dangerous, for newly qualified therapists (NQTs) to work straight away in private practice. Best and safe practice comes only from a measured trajectory from preceptorship period to generalist and onto developing and established specialist practice, that plots thresholds of tested competence and appraised skills. It is also a journey of life experience and cannot be rushed. It is enriching that many NQTs are mature students who bring life experience, and skills and training from complementary careers, into the SLT profession. We reiterate our central theme of this book: that you cannot teach and coach what you do not know and cannot embody and perform yourself, but with regular commitment to your vocal learning and understanding of vocal coaching, you can become the SLTs we need in the field *in time*. The current expansion in gender services and staff recruitment has seen a rise in appointments of inexperienced SLTs who find themselves out of their depth. This results both from pressures on recruiters to fill posts, and from a lack of adequate and experienced understanding of the skill profile needed to be a trans voicing specialist. This is far from acceptable in the delivery of on-point and effective voice work for our clients, and the antithesis of being of service and client-centred. We advocate urgently for a much greater shared understanding profession-wide of the suite of skills that defines and develops the trans-affirmative SLT, as we have aimed to set out throughout the key points of this book. The students of today are the new therapists of tomorrow, and the potential educators and supervisors of the future.

49 DOING THE WORK: AFFIRMATIONS AND LEARNING STATEMENTS

We are in the business of encouraging a therapeutic community of people who value trans lives and rights in all contexts and who foreground that value in their practice. We are a clinical community that recognises that trans and non-binary people have financial barriers to accessing private care and many limitations to accessing any care. We encourage vigilance in the reflectiveness and examination of our social and clinical privilege, cultural bias and vocal coaching competence. We centre the expertise and wisdom of lived experience and develop our skills through training, supervision and co-productive enterprise with trans and non-binary people. Look at Figure 9.1. Below are affirmations and learning statements we suggest – and hope – you keep in your heart, mind, body and practice as you enter and continue long into this field.

- **Trans cultural humility**
  - I meet my clients where they are, with respect, care and compassion, and foreground trans people's rights and expertise in their lives.
  - I engage in ongoing self-development so that my outlook, behaviours and practice align with respectful allyship, advocacy and activism.

Summary – The Trans-Affirmative SLT

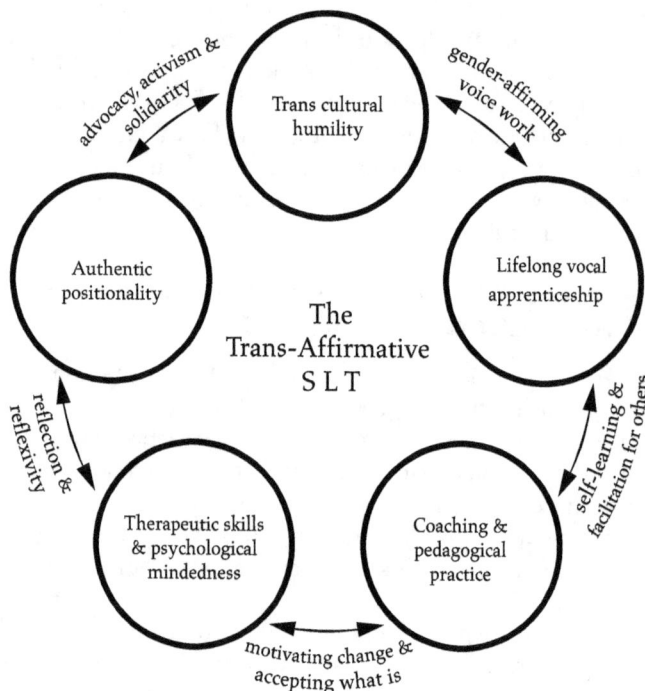

Figure 9.1 The Trans-Affirmative SLT

- I deeply believe that trans and non-binary people are experts in themselves and can only thrive and prosper when they live in accordance with their own sense of themselves.
- I deeply believe that there are no interventions that can or should aim to change gender identity or sexual orientation, and conversion therapy practices

are unethical, harmful, de-humanising, not supported by evidence and deeply transphobic.
- I dispense with fundamentally unhelpful conceptualisations of what is 'real' when it comes to people's sense of themselves in their gender identity and sexual orientation and identity.
- I stand with trans and non-binary people's right to live in congruence with their individual felt sense of gender, with freedom from restriction, aspersion, rejection, aggression, hate, violence and transphobia.
- I deeply believe that trans and non-binary people must have equitable access to the full spectrum of healthcare required to meet their needs and promote their well-being, irrespective of their gender identity or anatomy.
- I understand that some trans people may need access to psychological support in navigating aspects of physical and social transition, but mandatory psychotherapy for trans and non-binary people is not only inappropriate before any interventions, but is de-humanising and transphobic.
- I support trans and non-binary people to access care and explore gender identity without pressure or assumption of any particular outcome, and this includes and is particularly relevant to children and young people under the age of 16.
- I am sensitive to and respectful of trans and queer cultural practices, and open to new learning which centres community lived expertise.

- **Lifelong vocal apprenticeship**
  - I start with my own vocal awareness, and journey of development towards vocal conscious competence.
  - I recognise that I am always in vocal learning and apprenticeship, through and within novice to master craftsperson levels.
  - I aim for lived experience that recognises every day is a new day with my voice and vocal processing.

- I deeply believe and embody the compassion that every voice is unique, authentic and utterly personal.
- I commit to a creating a world of vocal belonging, not vocal othering.
- I commit to the lifelong journey, deepest understanding and felt sense of my own voice, its flexibilities, idiosyncrasies and imperfections which in time I offer up to the process of becoming a sensitive and effective voice coach.

- **Coaching and pedagogical practice**
  - I work and develop to provide voice therapy which is pedagogically ethical and of the highest integrity.
  - I enjoy the complexity of this work and give myself permission and time to develop.
  - I work from the outset towards my clients' vocal independence, and my own therapeutic and coaching redundancy, whether I work in socialised care or private practice.
  - I commit to undertaking training, supervision – including vocal supervision – and continuing professional development in voice and gender healthcare, to ensure I am equipped to provide effective, client-centred gender-affirming voice and communication therapy.

- **Therapeutic skills and psychological mindedness**
  - I work to develop and provide voice therapy which is therapeutically safe and clinically self-interrogated which centres empathy, respect, congruence, co-production, cultural humility and multidirectional learning.
  - I work towards becoming psychologically minded, sensitive to transference and countertransference, the human interactions of the Drama Triangle, and group process.
  - I undertake supervision and reflect on my practice which intersects therapeutic process, pedagogical practice and cultural humility.
  - I offer voice therapy that not only aims to alleviate gender dysphoria but enables trans and non-binary

people to experience significant comfort and gender euphoria in life.
- I endeavour to provide voice therapy sensitive to and respectful of a diversity of neurodivergence and access needs.
- **Authentic positionality**
  - I examine my implicit biases, and interrogate the privilege I wield as a clinician and therapist, knowing this is ongoing reflexive work.
  - I commit to seeking continuing cultural humility development from the trans and queer community.
  - I deeply believe that trans women are women, trans men are men and non-binary people are valid without question.
  - I continually reflect on my social privilege, my intersectional identities, my relationship to gender and cisheteronormativity and the influences of white supremacy, imperialism, capitalism and patriarchy.
  - I deeply believe that the diversity of gender identity is intrinsically part of the human experience and always has been.
  - I deeply believe that gender identity is an utterly individual and personally verifiable experience, deeply ingrained and intrinsic to who people are; it is neither decision nor lifestyle choice.
  - I condemn discrimination in all its forms, and aim to raise up marginalised people and communities.
  - I deeply believe that healthcare for trans and non-binary people must not be prohibited for reasons of personal finance or any protected characteristic.
  - I work to maximise and celebrate trans and non-binary people's autonomy in their voice and communication identities and in lives of trans joy.

50 AUTHOR DIALOGUE 'BE THE FUTURE'

Natasha: So, Matthew, we have set out, summarised in bite-size pieces, and discussed in some detail the concepts, debates, knowledge and skills that students and new and, in fact, established therapists need to be thinking about and reflecting on now and into the future. It's dynamic.

Matthew: Thanks, yes. So, how can we bring our discussions together to a close, Natasha? What are your words of encouragement and discernment for our readers – becoming skilled vocal pedagogues and therapists for the trans community?

Natasha: I would say that – this is complex work. This complexity may not be valued or fully acknowledged in the professional consciousness at the moment, and there may not be an understanding of the many competencies that are needed in this field, particularly in these times of aggressive culture wars and relentless de-humanising of trans identities.

Matthew: Yes, in these harsh times. And competencies in medical settings such as dysphagia management, laryngoscopy, tracheostomy, fiberoptic endoscopic evaluation of swallowing can be seen as more complex and more valuable somehow than complexities in trans voicing ...

Natasha: Yes, at first glance voice therapy may not seem to be complex in that way, but it is complex. It is complex in terms of therapists needing to work with implicit biases, the programming that we all carry, the work we have to do to look into ourselves to undo the 'damage' done to all of us as humans by the social programming and prejudice we all ingest, to develop finely tuned counselling skills and core conditions, to be culturally guided by we who are in the trans community in terms of specific practices and remembrances, to understand and use inclusive language, to have personal voice skill and know-how in voice coaching and teaching, so you can ethically guide trans people like me and many others. You need to be equipped with solution based approaches, mindfulness and compassion centred work which acknowledges the uniqueness of your individual trans clients and their intersectional identities and levels of marginalisation, and their authentic voices. And please collaborate with and respect trans community voice resources and expert practitioners who are more and more visible. Wow, that's a lot of work!

Matthew: It is but as we say, start building your skills brick by brick, step by step. You are different now as a result of reading this book, and thinking about the ideas we have put forward. We hope you return to these key points again and again as a reference to layering your depth of understanding, and to support your fledgling and accomplished practice.

Natasha: Yes, and despite the many complexities that define this field, trans voicing in all its glory, I would say because there *is* complexity, it can also be very enjoyable! So, enjoy it! This is *really important work* and it can feel really rewarding. It is really needed, really valuable work. So, I say – we both say – 'go for it!', don't we?

Matthew: Yes, we do! 'Go for it!' Thank you, Natasha, for your eloquence and wise words here and throughout all the writing and discussions.

Natasha: Thank you for this opportunity to share, hone and refine, Matthew, and thank you to our readers especially, for being and travelling with us. To quote the maxim that is at the heart of our work and journey, that simple but powerful statement of solidarity, 'we are in the boat together … '

APPENDIX OF RESOURCES

USEFUL TRANS ORGANISATIONS

AKT – the Albert Kennedy Trust is a LGBTQ+ homeless charity offering housing, training and advocacy. www.akt.org.uk

All About Trans – an organisation which aims to educate and change media representation of trans people. www.allabouttrans.org.uk

All Out – this is a movement worldwide seeking to build a world where no one sacrifices their freedom due to their identity. http://allout.org

Distinction – a group aiming to provide help to partners of trans people. www.distinctionsupport.org

Gendered Intelligence – a not-for-profit Community Interest Company working with trans community, specialising in youth projects and working with trans people under 21. www.genderedintelligence.co.uk

The Gender Identity Research and Education Society (GIRES) – aims to improve the lives of trans and non-binary people through policy and research and publishes a directory of groups in the UK supporting trans people. Tranzwiki www.gires.org.uk

IMAAN – LGBTQ Muslim charity in the UK. www.imaan.org.uk

LGBT Foundation – a charity in Manchester and community support for trans and non binary people, affiliated with the Indigo gender clinic. https://lgbtfoundation

Mermaids – an organisation leading to support trans and non-binary children and young people and their families. www.mermaidsuk.org.uk

Press for Change – established by Christine Burns and is an organisation expert in legal matters and the law related to trans people. www.pfc.org.uk

Scottish Trans Alliance – an organisation dedicated to improve the lives of trans and non-binary people in Scotland. www.scottishtrans.org

Spectra – an organisation offering health advocacy, counselling, peer mentoring and social groups for trans and non-binary people. https://spectra-london.org.uk/trans-services/

Stonewall – a key organisation campaigning for the rights of LBGTQ people (trans people since 2014). www.stonewall.org.uk

Terrence Higgins Trust – a charity dedicated to supporting the LGBTQ community with sexual health, HIV and mental health advice and counselling services. www.tht.org.uk

TransActual – an organisation highlighting the issues affecting trans and non-binary people in society publishing surveys and research. www.lgbtconsortium.org.uk/directory/trans-actural-uk

Trans London – a London-based support group run by Martha Dunkley for trans and non-binary people meeting at Gay's The Word bookshop. www.facebook.com/groups/TransLondon

Trans Media Watch – a charity working to improve media coverage and portrayal of trans and non-binary and intersex people. www.transmediawatch.org

Trans Unite – a directory of support and community groups for trans and non-binary people. www.transunite.co.uk

UNIQUE Transgender Network – a befriending and trans-led support group founded by Jenny-Anne Bishop OBE working in North Wales and West Cheshire. www.uniquetg.org.uk

GENDER SERVICES IN THE UK (INCLUDING GENDER IDENTITY CLINICS, GENDER SERVICES, AND PILOT CLINICS OF WHICH MORE ARE DUE TO BE CREATED)

Brackenburn Gender Identity Clinic
CMAGIC Gender Dysphoria Service
East of England Gender Service
Grampian Gender Identity Clinic
Highlands Gender Identity Clinic
Indigo Gender Service
Lothian Gender Identity Clinic
Northamptonshire Gender Identity Clinic
Northern Region Gender Dysphoria Service
Sandyford Gender Identity Service
Sussex Gender Service
The Leeds Gender Identity Service
The Nottingham Centre for Transgender Health
The Sheffield Gender Identity Clinic ('Porterbrook')
The Tavistock and Portman Gender Identity Clinic for Adults ('London GIC'/previously known as 'Charing Cross GIC')
The West of England Specialist Gender Identity Clinic ('The Laurels')
TransPlus
Welsh Gender Service

TRANS HEALTH ORGANISATIONS AND ASSOCIATIONS

The British Association of Gender Identity Specialists (BAGIS). https://bagis.co.uk
The European Professional Association of Transgender Health (EPATH). https://epath.eu
The World Professional Association of Transgender Health (WPATH). www.wpath.org

VOICE SPECIFIC TRAINING AND DEVELOPMENT

City Academy. www.city-academy.com/voice-training
The City Literary Institute. www.citylit.ac.uk/courses/performing-arts/voice-and-speech
Morrison Bone Prop. www.themorrisonboneprop.com
Royal Central School of Speech and Drama. www.cssd.ac.uk/courses/voice-studies-teaching-and-coaching-mamfa
Royal College of Speech and Language Therapists National Clinical Excellence Network Trans Voice. www.rcslt.org/speech-and-language-therapy/clinical-information/trans-voice/#section-4

COMMUNITY-LED TRANS VOICE WORK

Trans Choir London. https://londontranschoir.com
Trans Voice Training. www.transvoicetraining.co.uk
TransVoiceLessons. www.youtube.com/@TransVoiceLessons

DOCUMENTARIES AND TALKS

Campbell, X. (2021). *Making queer film: Campbell X – The coast is queer 2021*. www.youtube.com/watch?v=qwB-irHOjTw&t=201s
Preston, A. M., & TEDx Talks. (2018). *Effective allyship: A transgender take on intersectionality*. www.youtube.com/watch?v=3EcuDfDjUd8
Tellyjuice. (2018). *The second train*. https://vimeo.com/289072627
Trans Health Care Welsh Gender Service. www.youtube.com/watch?v=Ym1jWVdcWFs

BIBLIOGRAPHY

Alabanza T (2022) *None of the Above: Reflections on Life Beyond the Binary*. Edinburgh: Canongate.

Barker M-J & Iantaffi A (2019) *Life Isn't Binary: On Being Both, Beyond, and in-Between*. London: Jessica Kingsley Publishers.

Barker M-J & Ryan-Flood R (2023) 'The Gender Wars and Difficult Conversations about Trans,' in R Ryan-Flood, I Crowhursrt, A Skamballis & L James-Hawkins (Eds.) *Difficult Conversations in Feminism*. London: Routledge, pp. 11–26.

Barker M-J & Scheele J (2016) *Queer: A Graphic History*. London: Icon Books.

Barker M-J & Scheele J (2019) *Gender: A Graphic Guide*. London: Icon Books.

Berne E (2010) *Games People Play*. London: Penguin.

Berry C (1994) *Your Voice and How to Use It* (revised edn). London: Virgin Books.

Bockting W, Miner MH, Swinburne Romine RE, Dolezal C, Robinson B, 'Bean' E, Rosser BRS & Coleman E (2020) 'The Transgender Identity Survey. A Measure of Internalised Transphobia,' *LGBT Health*, 7(1), 15–27.

Bornstein K (2013) *My New Gender Workbook*. New York: Routledge.

Boston J (2018) *Voice: Readings in Theatre Practice*. London: Palgrave

Burns C (2019) *Trans Britain: Our Journey from the Shadows*. London: Unbound.

Campbell P, Constantino S & Simpson S (2019) *Stammering Pride and Prejudice: Difference not Defect*. Guilford: J & R Press.

Choudrey S (2022) *Supporting Trans People of Colour: How to Make Your Practice Inclusive*. London: Jessica Kingsley Publishers.

Crenshaw K (1989) 'Demarginalizing the Intersection of Race and Sex: A Black Feminist Critique of Antidiscrimination Doctrine, Feminist Theory and Antiracist Politics,' *University of Chicago Legal Forum*, 1989(1), Article 8.

Denborough D (2014) *Retelling the Stories of Our Lives.* New York: W.W. Norton & Company.

de Shazer S (2012) *More than Miracles: The State of Art of Solution-Focused Brief Therapy* (2nd edn). New York: Routledge.

Faye S (2021) *The Transgender Issue.* London: Penguin.

Fausto-Sterling A (2012) *Sex/Gender: Biology in a Social World.* London: Routledge.

Fisher O & Fisher F (2021) *Trans Survival Workbook.* London: Jessica Kingsley Publishers.

Gilbert P (2015) *The Compassionate Mind: A New Approach to Life's Challenges.* London: Robinson.

Gratton FV (2019) *Supporting Transgender Autistic Youth and Adults: A Guide for Professionals and Families.* London: Jessica Kingsley Publishers.

HMSO (2004) Gender Recognition Act.

HMSO (2005) The Gender Recognition (Disclosure of Information (England, Wales and Northern Ireland) Order 2005HMSO (2010). The Equality Act.

hooks b (2000) *Feminist Theory: From Margin to Center.* London: Pluto Press.

Iantaffi A (2020) *Gender Trauma: Healing Cultural, Social, and Historical Gendered Trauma.* London: Jessica Kingsley Publishers.

Iantaffi A & Barker M-J (2018) *How to Understand Your Gender: A Practical Guide for Exploring Who You Are.* London: Jessica Kingsley.

Iantaffi A, Barker M-J, van Anders S & Scheele J (2018) *Mapping Your Sexuality: From Sexual Orientation to Sexual Configurations Theory.* www.rewriting-the-rules.com/wp-content/uploads/2018/08/MappingYourSecuality.pdf.

James S & Brumfit S (2018) *Applying Psychological Ideas in Speech and Language Therapy.* Guildford: J&R Press.

Kabat-Zinn J (2016) *Mindfulness for Beginners: Reclaiming the Present Moment and Your Life.* Boulder: Sounds True.

Karpman SB (1968) 'Fairy Tales and Script Drama Analysis,' *Transactional Analysis Bulletin,* 26(7), 39–43.

Karpman SB (2014) *A Game Free Life: The Definitive Book on the Drama Triangle and the Compassion Triangle by the Originator and Author.* San Francisco: Drama Triangle Productions.

Lester CN (2017) *Trans Like Me: A Journey For All of Us.* London: Hachette.

Lorimer S & Vincent B (2022) 'The Rationale for a Collaborative Deconstruction of a Gender Assessment Protocol,' Presented at the 7th Scientific Symposium of the British Association of Gender Identity Specialists (BAGIS), Liverpool 16–17 June, 2022.

Manning M (2022) *README.txt: A Memoir*. New York: Farrar, Straus & Giroux.

Marshall K (2020) 'The Gender Binary is a Tool of White Supremacy: a Brief History of Gender Expansiveness and how Colonialism Slaughtered it,' *Medium*. aninjusticemag.com/the-gender-binary-is-a-tool-of-white-supremacy-db89d0bc9044 [accessed 10.10.2023].

Meyer IH (1995) 'Minority Stress and Mental Health in Gay Men,' *Journal of Health and Social Behavior*, 36(1), 38.

Miles L (2020) *Transgender Resistance: Socialism and the Fight for Trans Liberation*. London: Bookmarks.

Mills M & Pert S (2024) *Working with Trans Voice*. Abingdon: Routledge.

Mills M & Stoneham G (2017) *The Voice Book for Trans and Non-binary People: A Practical Guide to Creating and Sustaining Authentic Voice and Communication*. London: Jessica Kingsley Publishers.

Mills M & Stoneham G (2021) *Voice and Communication Therapy with Trans and Non-Binary People: Sharing the Clinical Space*. London: Jessica Kingsley Publishers.

Mock J (2017) *Surpassing Certainty*. New York: Atria.

Morrison A (2022) *The Moment of Speech: Creative Articulation for Actors*. London: Methuen.

Pearce R (2018) *Understanding Trans Health*. Bristol: Policy Press.

Preston AM (2020) The Anatomy of Transmisogynoir. https://www.harpersbazaar.com/culture/features/a33614214/ashlee-marie-preston-transmisogynoir-essay/

Richards C & Barker M (2013) *Sexuality and Gender for Mental Health Professionals: A Practical Guide*. London: Sage.

Richards C & Barrett J (2021) *Trans and Non-Binary Gender Healthcare*. Cambridge: Cambridge University Press.

Roche J (2020a) *Trans Power: Own Your Gender*. London: Jessica Kingsley Publishers

Roche J (2020b) *Gender Explorers: Our Stories of Growing Up Trans and Changing the World*. London: Jessica Kingsley Publishers.

Rogers CR (1989) 'The Necessary and Sufficient Conditions of Therapeutic Personality Change,' *TACD Journal*, 17(1), 53–65. https://doi.org/10.1080/1046171x.1989.12034347.

Rogers CR (2004) *On Becoming a Person: A Therapist's View of Psychotherapy*. London: Constable & Robinson.

Scarrone Bonhomme L, Davies S & Beattie M (2023) *Gender Affirming Therapy*. Maidenhead: Open University Press.

Shlasko D (2017) *Trans Allyship Workbook: Building Skills to Support Trans People in Our Lives*. Madison: Think Again Training.

Steinhauer K, Klimmek MM & Estill J (2017) *The Estill Voice Model: Theory and Translation*. Pittsburgh, KS: Estill Voice International.

Titze IR & Verdolini Abbott K (2012) *Vocology: The Science and Practice of Voice Habilitation*. Salt Lake City, UT: Utah National Center for Voice and Speech.

Trans Lives Survey (2021) London. www.transactual.org.uk

Verdolini Abbott K (2008) *Lessac-Madsen Resonant Voice Therapy*. San Diego, CA: Plural Publishing.

Vincent B (2018) *Transgender Health: A Practitioner's Guide to Binary and Non-Binary Trans Patient Care*. London: Jessica Kingsley Publishers.

Vincent B (2020) *Non-binary Genders: Navigating Communities, Identities, and Healthcare*. Bristol: Policy Press.

White M (2007) *Maps of Narrative Practice*. New York: W.W. Norton & Co.

World Professional Association of Transgender Health (WPATH) (2020) *Standards of Care. Version 8*. Minneapolis, MN: WPATH.

INDEX

Page numbers in **bold** refer to tables; those in *italics* refer to figures.

accent 26, 88
accomplice 52
activist 52
adaptation 58–9, 96, 107–9, 112, 114
advocate 52
agender 17
agreeing sounds 112
Alabanza, Travis 22
ally 52, 55–6
allyship 51, 55, 121
androgens 5
androgynous 9, 17, 112
ask etiquette 51, 53
assertiveness 96
assigned female at birth (AFAB) 7, 15, 17, 19, **20**
assigned male at birth (AMAB) 7, 15, 17, 19, **20**
assumptions 11, 13, 28, 34, 46, 53, 98
authenticity 32, 59, 66; vocal 68–9, 74
autonomy 58–9, 125; body 64, 115
awakening and extending 89

Barker, Meg-John 71
belonging 5, 6, 25, 32, 56, 74, 97; vocal: 71, 96, 124
bi-gender 18, 62
biofeedback 73

bright tone 109–10
Burns, Christine 22, 130

Challenger 78, 82–3
Choudrey, Sabah 22, 48–9
chromosomes 5, 7
circle of: all life concern 57; existential concern 25; human concern 68
cis-centric 36, 39, 82
cis-temic 95
cisgender: 31, 34, 45; bias 40; privilege 45; vocal superiority 31
cisheteronormativity 6, 13, 18, 27, 125
cisnormative 97, 106
co-creator 82–3
code-switches 71, 74, 113
cognitive-process: consonance 96, 107, 109–10, 112; dissonance 109
colonialism 11
coming out 31, 33
Compassion Focused Therapy 80
congruence 64, 78–9, 123–4
consent **20**, 23, 38, 117
core conditions 79–80, 83, **126**
counselling skills 79–80, 83
countertransference 78–9, 94, 124
cricothyroid approximation **61**

cultural: competence 12; humility 5, 12–14, 51, 66, 119, 121, 124–5

deadname 16, 36
dominant culture 7, 9, 12
Dunkley, Martha 130

empathy 9, 52, 56, 78–9, 83, 124
enby 17
Estill Voice Training 86

Facilitator 82, 95
Fa'afafine 10
Fisher, Owl and Fox 14–15, 48

gate-keeping 22
Gender Incongruence 17, 21, 59
genderfluid 18
genderfuck 18
genderqueer 6, 17
genital reconstruction surgery **61**
gestural cueing 109
Gillick competence 44
glottoplasty **61**
Gratton, Finn 22
grounding and aligning 88

haptic 87
hate crime 28, 43, 46
Hijra 10
High-Bright-Thin 85, 98, 105, *106*
hormone replacement therapy (HRT) 34, 58–9, **60**, 62, 64
humming 107, 109

ICD 17, 21–2
imposter syndrome 66, 71, 73, 85, 90, 92, 95–7, 107
intersectionality 6, 6, 11, 49,
intersex people 7, 44, 130

'in the boat together' 79, 83, 127
intoning into speaking 107, 110

Jam, Mila 48
jaw shake 112
Journey of Voice Development 116

Launch-Express-Land *106*, 107–9
Lester, CN 22
Low-Chest-Thick 85, 98, 110, *111*

Machi 10
macro and microaggressions 17, 43, 46
Manning, Chelsea 22
Mahu 10
mindfulness 80, 115
misgendering 17, 45–6, 54
misogyny 32
Mock, Janet 22
motor learning 73, 85, 93, 95, 103
multiplicity of gender 3

Nambiar, Kate 59
Narrative Therapy (NT) 68, 80, 116
neopronouns 54
neurodivergence 125
neurodiversity 6, 26, 125

oestrogen **60**, 62, 102

paradox of change 69
paraphrasing 79
passaggio 112, 115
pathologisation 6, 67
patriarchy 11, 40, 125
perfect piano keyboard app 104
Persecutor 82, 94
person-centred 73, 79

pitch launching 98, 105, 108, 112, 115, 117; resting 98, 104, 108, 113
playing and articulating 89
plurality 2, 66, 84
positionality 5, 25, 56, 77, 98, 119, 125
praxis 73, 114
presence 96
privilege: cis 6, 18; clinical 13, 70, 121
pronouns 9, 17, 30–1, 34-5, 49, 53–5, 57, 98–9
psychological contact 78, 79
pure exercise 95–6, 107, 109, 110, 112, 113–14

quick win warm-ups 114

relational voice 66, 71
Rescuer 82, 95
resonance contrast 107
Rashid, Tina 59
Resonant Voice Therapy 86
Roche, Juno 21, 22, 41
Rodriguez, Michaela Jae 48

scaffolding 94, 108
semi-tone 113, 115
sex/gender 11–12, 15
shamanic 10
shame 31, 45
singing **61**, 112, 115
Solution-Focused Therapy 80
somatic 87
Standards of Care 35
sternum hook up 112
stretching and releasing 89
summarising 79, 98

testosterone 8, **60**, 62, 111, 113
The Drama Triangle 78, 80, 94, 124
The Second Train 132
thinking sound 107, 109
third gender 10
thyroid: prominence 3; chondroplasty **61**; notch **61**
Trans Day of Remembrance (TDoR) 43, 47–8
Trans Day of Visibility (TDoV) 43, 48
trans joy 43, 47–8, 55, 125
transfeminine 19, 33, **60–1**
transference 78–9, 94, 124
transmasculine 19, 32, 40, **60–1**
transmisogynoir 31–2
trauma-informed 16, 45, 95
twang quality 90
Two Spirit 10

unconditional positive regard 42, 78, 80

Victim 82, 94–5
vocal fold: length 5; thickening **60**; weight 72, 96, 98, 105, 113
vocal: authenticity 68–9, 74, 92; collaboration 71, 74; home 68–71; journeying 66–7, 74; othering 96–7, 124; pedagogy 72, 74; profile 69, 113; plurality 74
voicing and resonating 89

White, Michael 68, 116

X, Campbell 48

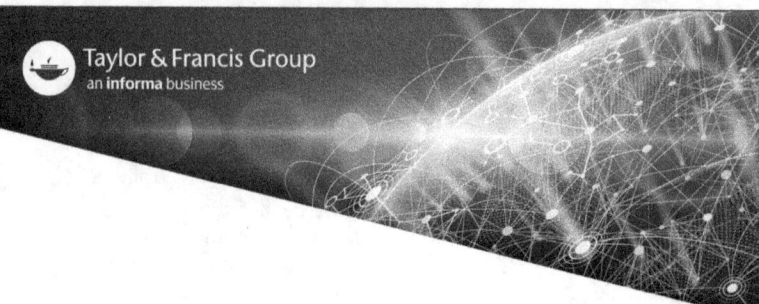

For Product Safety Concerns and Information please contact our EU representative GPSR@taylorandfrancis.com
Taylor & Francis Verlag GmbH, Kaufingerstraße 24, 80331 München, Germany

www.ingramcontent.com/pod-product-compliance
Lightning Source LLC
Chambersburg PA
CBHW051749230426
43670CB00012B/2209